ABOUT THE AUTHOR

Deepak Chopra is the bestselling author of twenty-five books, including *Ageless Body, Timeless Mind* and *The Path to Love*. He is the Director of Educational Programmes at The Chopra Center for Well Being in La Jolla, California.

Other books by Deepak Chopra

Creating Health
Return of the Rishi
Quantum Healing
Perfect Health
Unconditional Life
Ageless Body, Timeless Mind
Perfect Weight
Journey into Healing
Creating Affluence
The Seven Spiritual Laws of Success
The Return of Merlin
Restful Sleep
Perfect Digestion
The Way of the Wizard
Overcoming Addictions
Raid on the Inarticulate
The Path to Love
The Seven Spiritual Laws for Parents
The Love Poems of Rumi (edited by Deepak Chopra; translated by Deepak Chopra and Fereydoun Kia)
Healing the Heart
Everyday Immortality
The Lords of the Light
On the Shores of Eternity
How to Know God
The Chopra Centre Herbal Handbook

DEEPAK CHOPRA

BOUNDLESS ENERGY

the complete mind-body programme for overcoming chronic fatigue

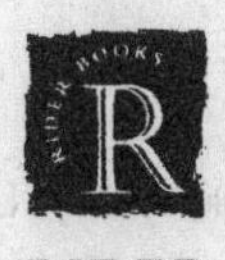

RIDER

LONDON · SYDNEY · AUCKLAND · JOHANNESBURG

15

Published in 1995 by Rider, an imprint of Ebury Publishing
This edition published by Rider in 2001
First published in the USA by Harmony Books, a division of Crown Publishers, Inc., in 1995

Ebury Publishing is a Random House Group company

The Random House Group Limited Reg. No. 954009

Addresses for companies within the Random House Group can be found at www.randomhouse.co.uk

A CIP catalogue record for this book is available from the British Library

Designed by Lauren Dong

ISBN 9780712602945

This book gives non-specific, general advice and should not be relied on as a substitue for proper medical consultation. The author and publisher cannot accept responsibility for illness arising out of the failure to seek medical advice from a doctor.

Printed and bound in Great Britain by Clays Ltd, St Ives plc

Contents

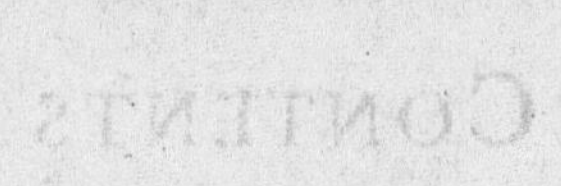

Contents

Boundless Energy

1

Fatigue, Energy, and the Quantum Mechanical Body

Fatigue is the absence of physical, intellectual, and emotional energy, and chronic fatigue is a prolonged absence of this energy. As someone living in contemporary Western society, however, you probably have no need for a definition of fatigue. You're likely to be quite familiar with the problem already. In fact, there's an excellent chance that you're living with chronic fatigue right now.

Despite the fact that fatigue is widespread in modern life, it really is a unique phenomenon when seen in the context of nature as a whole. After all, nature abounds with energy and purposeful activity. Birds awaken early, sing, tirelessly build their nests, and gather food for their young; squirrels bound up tree trunks and jump from branch to branch; and in spring, the grass and the flowers almost seem to leap from the earth with exuberance and vitality.

This astonishing energy is present not only in the biological world but in the physical universe as well. Waves crash against the shore; rivers rush toward the sea with incredible power; the wind howls, pushing everything before it; the earth spins on its axis and circles the sun at incredible speed; and the sun itself is continually producing unimaginable amounts of heat and light. Physicists tell us that the universe is nothing other than one dynamic, pulsating field of overwhelming energy.

It's puzzling, isn't it? With so much energy throughout nature, how can anyone possibly feel fatigued? Why is fatigue a daily experience for millions of people? Why, for many of them, is it the dominant experience of their lives?

The discrepancy between the prevalence of chronic fatigue in our society and the abundant energy in the natural world creates a troubling paradox. But it can also provide an important clue for finding the real answer to chronic fatigue. In this book you'll learn many techniques for reestablishing the connection between yourself and nature; more specifically, you'll learn how to uncover the natural sources of energy that are already within you.

Before going into the solutions, let's look more closely at the problem of fatigue in our society and get some idea of its scope.

Fatigue is one of the most common complaints that people bring to doctors. A recent study published in the *Journal of the American Medical Association* found that 24 percent of patients who were randomly surveyed in the waiting room of a general medical clinic complained of chronic fatigue. Women reported a higher rate of fatigue than men—28 percent were fatigued compared to 19 percent of men—but the incidence in men was still almost one in five.

While there's no doubt that fatigue is a constant presence in the lives of millions of Americans, it is also one of the most elusive complaints for a physician to evaluate, and only rarely can a definitive cause be isolated. This is not to suggest that you shouldn't have a medical checkup if you're experiencing persistent, deep fatigue that has lasted for several weeks—there may be a clear-cut, easily treatable cause such as anemia, a thyroid problem, hepatitis, diabetes, mononucleosis, kidney problems, or another chronic health disorder. I recommend a physical exam to rule out these possible causes, but I also want to emphasize that for the overwhelming majority of people complaining of chronic fatigue, no specific physical cause can be discovered. Indeed, this may be the single most important finding in all the many studies that examined the problem.

For the purposes of this book, chronic fatigue means a noticeable lack of energy that has been present for one month or more. This is very different from acute fatigue, which is usually brought on by the demands of specific situations, such as cramming for an exam or rushing to meet a deadline at work. Acute fatigue generally disappears with the passage of time and some extra rest. People who are chronically fatigued continue to feel tired no matter how much rest they get. In fact, it is quite common for chronically fatigued people to feel tired immediately upon waking up in the morning, and even *more* tired after they get up and about. Clearly, sleep alone is not sufficient to solve the problem of chronic fatigue.

To sum up, then, we can define chronic fatigue as fatigue that has lasted for at least one month, that is present every day or almost every day, and that is not cured by sleep or rest.

THE MIND/BODY CONNECTION AND CHRONIC FATIGUE SYNDROME

Despite the widespread incidence of chronic fatigue throughout the population, the magnitude of its impact on normal life is probably underestimated by many people. Studies have shown that chronic fatigue can be every bit as debilitating as serious medical disorders such as untreated thyroid disease or a recent heart attack. This is even more remarkable in light of the fact that the overwhelming majority of people with chronic fatigue do not have a clear physical cause for their problem.

In the absence of such a cause, it has become clear that most chronic fatigue is strongly influenced by emotional and psychological factors. For example, studies have found that up to 80 percent of chronically fatigued people score higher than normal on psychological tests of depression or anxiety. This brings up a very important idea—the mind/body connection—which will be a central theme of this book. Your mind and your emotions can be major sources of energy or major wasters of it, and the choice is entirely yours. We will explore this concept in detail in the pages that follow.

Before going any further, however, it's important to mention a subgroup of people who have an especially severe version of fatigue which has come to be known as Chronic Fatigue Syndrome. CFS is a specific disorder that was first recognized medically in the mid-1980s. Although there is currently no firm agreement among health care professionals regarding the cause of the problem, there is evidence that suggests viral infection and malfunction of the immune system may be involved.

Data from the federal Center for Disease Control and Prevention indicates that true Chronic Fatigue Syndrome affects between 100,000 and 250,000 adults nationwide. These people experience a type of fatigue that is sufficiently intense and persistent to reduce normal daily activities by at least 50 percent for a minimum of six months, and it also includes specific physiological symptoms that distinguish CFS from a simple lack of energy. CFS patients often sleep twelve hours a day or more, yet they have great difficulty performing routine tasks, due to exhaustion. Individuals with the usual kind of chronic fatigue can generally manage to push themselves through their daily activities, but people with Chronic Fatigue Syndrome are truly disabled by their disorder. CFS also commonly includes physical symptoms such as low-grade fever, recurrent sore throat, painful lymph nodes, muscle aches or weakness, joint pains, and headaches. Sleep seems unrefreshing, and there may also be problems with concentration and short-term memory.

If you have symptoms that suggest Chronic Fatigue Syndrome, you should see a doctor for medical evaluation.

THE TRUE SOURCES OF CHRONIC FATIGUE

By now we recognize that chronic fatigue is a very common problem that can manifest itself as a moderately severe impediment to the enjoyment of life, or that can be genuinely devastating when it assumes the form of Chronic Fatigue Syndrome. But the solution to the problem is always the same: *more energy.*

Specifically, the remedy for chronic fatigue—and the basis for achieving a more fulfilling experience of life in general—lies in the ability to tap into the unlimited natural field of energy that surrounds us at every moment. Einstein revealed that every atom in the universe contains an enormous amount of power, and contemporary physics continues to demonstrate that everything in the universe comes into being through fluctuations in a *unified field* of energy and intelligence, which is the very foundation of nature. In other words, a single source of energy underlies everything, and it is from this source that all the phenomena of the universe are brought into existence. As human beings, we are simply localized concentrations of energy and intelligence in the universal field. The intelligence and energy that flows through our bodies is the same as that which governs the universe. We and everything around us are part of a continuum with nature.

All this becomes clear when we consider the atoms that compose the human body. Quantum physics has shown that the atoms themselves are not solid, irreducible objects. They are made up of subatomic particles—protons, neutrons, and electrons—which whirl around each other at lightning speeds. And within each atom the distances between these subatomic particles are proportionately as great as the distances between stars and galaxies. This means that the human body is proportionately as void as intergalactic space.

From a physicist's point of view, even subatomic particles are not solid, tangible objects. Rather, they too are fluctuations of energy that have taken on a material form. Einstein said that matter is really nothing but energy cloaked in a different form, and the great physicists of the 1920s and 1930s confirmed that every physical particle is ultimately a form of energy vibration called a "wave function." This revelation—that matter is actually a form of wave vibration—is called "wave-particle duality" in quantum physics.

These insights from the most advanced branches of modern science can provide us with an entirely new understanding of our bodies. Beyond its material form, the body is really a pulsating, dynamic field of energy. The individual particles that make up the body are energy vibrations within the larger, universal field. Underlying our material being there exists what might be called a "quantum mechanical body," which is pure process, pure energy, and pure intelligence. Since the quantum mechanical body determines what the material body will be like, it is in the quantum mechanical body that we'll find the origins of chronic fatigue, and also the keys for eliminating it.

While most of us (with the exception of quantum physicists) think of the body as something solid and physical, we also think of the mind as insubstantial, nonmaterial, ghostlike. As long as this perceived dichotomy remains, it will be difficult to understand how mind and body can possibly interact with each other. But now the relationship between them is precisely the focus of a new area of science known as mind/body medicine, which is offering exciting solutions to some of the most difficult and frustrating problems in contemporary health care.

Once you understand that the apparently material structure of the body is really nothing other than pure energy, it becomes clear that thought and matter are fundamentally alike. From the point of view of quantum physics, there is not much difference between fluctuations of thought arising within the unified field and the wave vibrations that give rise to the particles that make up the human body. In short, your thoughts are quantum events, subtle vibrations of the field, that have a profound influence on all the functions of your body.

Recent research at the National Institutes of Health has gained important insights into the relationship between the mind and the physical body. It has become clear that an entire category of chemicals, called neuropeptides, is produced by the brain every time a thought or feeling occurs. The type of neuropeptide produced corresponds to the quality of thought or feeling that has taken place. And most important, these neuropeptides are not confined to the brain or nervous system. Receptors to neuropeptides have been found throughout the digestive system, the heart, lungs, kidneys, and in the immune system as well. This indicates that neuropeptides have a powerful effect on all physiological processes, including energy production and immunity.

Once we begin to grasp the mind/body connection—that is, how thoughts and emotions affect the body—we can begin to understand the causes of chronic fatigue. We can understand why research has shown that chronic fatigue patients generally do not have specific physical problems, but tend to have higher than normal levels of depression and anxiety. This is a crucial point: it appears to be a deficit in the emotional and mental life of an individual that robs the body of energy and produces chronic fatigue. This energy drain is a function of the mind/body connection, and it is governed by chemicals produced in the brain.

At any moment, your perceived energy level is the product of a large number of variables, such as the quality of your food and digestion, the temperature of the air around you, your thoughts and emotions, and many more. But the level of basic vitality you experience in daily life is determined by the quality of your connection to the unified field of energy that surrounds you. This connection controls the infusion of energy and intelligence into all your bodily systems, and it governs how well your physiological processes are working at every moment.

With this quantum mechanical viewpoint as a foundation, I am going to offer some rules that can help you experience pure energy rather than chronic fatigue. We will call these rules Primary Energy Principles, or PEPs, and in each chapter of this book new ones will be introduced. As you read, I suggest that you keep a pen and paper handy in order to write down the PEPs as you encounter them. This will focus your attention and help you to commit the PEPs to memory.

The first one explains why learning these principles will be of great benefit to your health.

> PEP 1. Knowledge has organizing power. Through the mind/body connection, knowledge affects the body and creates health.

Quite literally, knowledge can heal, and according to mind/body medicine, knowledge is the greatest healer of all. Therefore if you write down each of the PEPs and take them to heart, the effect can actually be like a medicinal prescription for your mind/body physiology. The neurochemicals that will become structured in your system will help to nourish, heal, and revitalize you in a very real and very profound way.

Here are four more PEPs:

> PEP 2. Energy is natural to life. The fact that unlimited energy is always present and available in the unified field is the most basic truth of nature.

> PEP 3. Energy flows naturally from the unified field to the mind/body system. Fatigue results from blocks or imbalances in this natural flow.

PEP 4. Blocks or imbalances in the mind/body system develop when harmony with nature has been disrupted.

PEP 5. A balanced mind/body system allows energy to flow easily from nature. Therefore the key to eliminating chronic fatigue and having abundant energy is *balance.*

Our first five PEPs contain important information about energy and fatigue, and they also serve to illuminate the relationship of any individual to the surrounding universe. PEP number 5, for example, refers to balance, which will be the key principle of this book. Balance is the goal of all the techniques you'll be learning, and it's a word that should be understood in a holistic way. Ideally, balance means complete integration of physical and spiritual components in every area of your experience.

In the chapters that follow, you'll learn techniques for creating balance in four areas: your body, your mind, your behavior, and your environment.

The first technique, which is a mind/body method for reducing fatigue, is called "energy tracking." Very simply, this involves making yourself more aware of the level of energy you experience throughout the day. It derives from our first Primary Energy Principle—*knowledge has organizing power.* You can actually begin solving the problem of chronic fatigue merely by increasing your awareness of your own feelings.

Why should you track energy rather than fatigue? The answer lies in our sixth PEP, which is called the Principle of the Second Element. Please write it down:

PEP 6. The Principle of the Second Element states that the ultimate solution to any problem is not on the level of the problem itself. Rather, the solution appears when a second element is introduced that is opposite to the problem.

To clarify this principle, let me offer an anecdotal illustration. People in a dark room may perceive that the darkness is a hindrance. Because of the darkness, they can't see what they're doing and they're constantly bumping into each other. They experience all sorts of difficulties and they simply can't enjoy life. But perhaps an intelligent group of people in the room will come together to think about how to solve the problem of darkness. They might form a committee to investigate its possible causes. They might try to diagnose various types and forms of darkness, and they might imagine all sorts of ways to treat it and eliminate it. Vast amounts of energy could be devoted to solving the problem of darkness on the level of the problem itself.

However, in the midst of all this analysis, one person might accidentally stumble against a switch on the wall, and the room would be filled with light. In an instant, the darkness is gone! It would suddenly become clear that darkness was not the problem. The real problem was the absence of a second element—in this case, light. In fact, the darkness itself had no reality except in a negative sense; it was merely the absence of a positive element.

Similarly, fatigue itself is not a problem. Fatigue is merely the absence of a positive force, which is energy. According to the principle of the Second Element, the solution to the problem of fatigue can be achieved by focusing on energy. For this reason, all the techniques and principles that follow will be oriented toward enhancing energy in the mind/body system. Instead of becoming fascinated by the darkness, we'll concentrate on bringing in some light.

To become aware of the ebbs and flows of your energy every twenty-four hours, use the Energy Tracking Chart provided in this chapter. On the chart, you should note the energy levels you experience at three important points during the day. The first of these key moments occurs shortly after you wake up, the second is in the late afternoon around 4:00 P.M., and the last is in the evening at 8:00 P.M.

When you rate your energy, simply sit quietly and let your awareness encompass your whole body. Allow yourself a few minutes to focus on this in a setting where you're not likely to be interrupted. It may help to close your eyes and to breathe slowly and evenly. When you're ready, make a mental appraisal of your energy level and then enter it on the chart. In the "comments" section, you should mention any activities or experiences that may have affected your energy.

ENERGY TRACKING CHART

Stop and measure your level of energy at three key times during the day: shortly after you wake up in the morning, in the late afternoon at around 4:00 P.M., and in the evening at around 8:00 P.M.

To determine your level of energy, sit quietly and let your awareness be on your whole body. Then mentally note your energy level, using a scale of 0 to 10. Circle the number on the scale that most accurately describes your energy level.

0 = No energy, complete fatigue
5 = Equal amounts of fatigue and energy
10 = Complete energy and vitality, without any trace of fatigue

At the end of the week, connect the circles to show the general trend of your energy levels.

ENERGY LEVEL

Sunday			Monday			Tuesday			Wednesday			Thursday			Friday			Saturday		
AM	PM	PM	AM	PM	PM	AM	PM	PM	AM	PM	PM	AM	PM	PM	AM	PM	PM	AM	PM	PM
10	10	10	10	10	10	10	10	10	10	10	10	10	10	10	10	10	10	10	10	10
9	9	9	9	9	9	9	9	9	9	9	9	9	9	9	9	9	9	9	9	9
8	8	8	8	8	8	8	8	8	8	8	8	8	8	8	8	8	8	8	8	8
7	7	7	7	7	7	7	7	7	7	7	7	7	7	7	7	7	7	7	7	7
6	6	6	6	6	6	6	6	6	6	6	6	6	6	6	6	6	6	6	6	6
5	5	5	5	5	5	5	5	5	5	5	5	5	5	5	5	5	5	5	5	5
4	4	4	4	4	4	4	4	4	4	4	4	4	4	4	4	4	4	4	4	4
3	3	3	3	3	3	3	3	3	3	3	3	3	3	3	3	3	3	3	3	3
2	2	2	2	2	2	2	2	2	2	2	2	2	2	2	2	2	2	2	2	2
1	1	1	1	1	1	1	1	1	1	1	1	1	1	1	1	1	1	1	1	1
0	0	0	0	0	0	0	0	0	0	0	0	0	0	0	0	0	0	0	0	0

By using the chart to increase your awareness of what your body is experiencing, you can begin to eliminate the imbalances that are the basis of chronic fatigue. The chart will also provide a permanent written record of your progress as you begin applying the other techniques described in this book. You'll be able to see at a glance how fatigue is progressively replaced by energy as balance is restored to your system.

Remember: The key to overcoming fatigue and to living life with energy, zest, and fulfillment is balance. By living in harmony with the universe around you and with the universe within you, you can experience an infusion of energy beyond anything you might have imagined.

2

Your Unique Mind/Body Constitution

The universe is an infinite reservoir of unimaginable energy—and you are an expression of that energy. The same power that spins the planets around the sun resides within every human being, and it is abundantly available within you. It is present in every cell of your body and energizes your entire physiological system. Our goal in this book is to reestablish your contact with this latent reserve of unlimited biological energy, to make it fully accessible to you in everyday life.

As we saw in chapter 1, the secret to contacting your inner energy is the creation of *balance*. But in order to achieve this balance, you must grasp some important information about your own individual mind/body system.

From birth until death, each one of us has his or her own unique constitution, which is constantly expressing itself in dozens of mental and physical attributes. And all these characteristics, of course, are expressions of the same underlying reality—they are all quantum fluctuations in the same unified field. We can call this totality of mental and physical characteristics our "bodymind." Knowing the basic elements of your individual bodymind is the first all-important step in learning to create balance.

The concepts in this chapter and in those that follow are derived from the most recent scientific advances in Western medicine and also from the Indian tradition of Ayurveda, the oldest system of health-related knowledge in the world. Ayurveda—which in Sanskrit means "science of life"—is the most comprehensive system of mind/body medicine ever devised. It offers not only a great wealth of theoretical knowledge, but also practical techniques for achieving better health. The mind/body approaches of Ayurveda have been clinically verified in the treatment of hundreds of health concerns, from the common cold to cancer, and have proven extremely helpful in eliminating the problem of chronic fatigue.

It is an unfortunate fact that conventional medicine tends to pay more attention to differences among diseases than to those among people. Ayurveda, however, recognizes that the distinctive features of each individual are crucial to creating, improving, and preserving human health. Evidence for this is all around us. Who has not noticed how, on a cool autumn day, some people will be dressed in overcoats, scarves, and gloves, as if it were already winter, while others are wearing short-sleeved shirts, as if summer had never ended? In a similar way, there are people who can eat huge amounts of food, digest it easily, and then get hungry again two or three hours later—while others are able to eat only much smaller quantities, have difficulty with digestion, and don't want to eat again for many hours. These differences in basic physiological characteristics lead directly and inescapably to the recognition that there are different mind/body types.

The same kinds of variations that are apparent in people's eating habits are also displayed in their levels of energy and fatigue. We've all encountered individuals who seem to have unlimited energy resources. They're able to wake up early, perhaps with relatively little sleep; they're dynamically active all day; they go out in the evening or perhaps continue with their work; and they do this day after day without ever seeming fatigued. Other people—and perhaps you are in this category—feel tired after managing simple everyday tasks, or they may even become exhausted just by starting off the day. Clearly, different levels of metabolism give rise to different patterns of energy production. Each of us has his or her own "biological individuality," which Ayurveda describes in terms of psychophysiological types.

In this book, for the sake of simplicity, we'll refer to individual constitutional types as "body types," although they definitely involve both mental and physical characteristics. The Ayurvedic term for body type is *prakriti,* a Sanskrit word that literally means "nature." Your Ayurvedic body type is nothing less than your own individual nature; it's like a blueprint that outlines the innate tendencies that have been built into your system. Learning about your Ayurvedic body type provides important information for reawakening your body's inner intelligence and for reestablishing a connection with your internal energy. To define the different body types Ayurveda focuses on the junction point between the physical and the spiritual. This is a fascinating area of interest, and a crucial one for understanding chronic fatigue.

We saw in chapter 1 that the mind and the body do meet. Every event in the mind produces a corresponding event in the body; a chemical reaction takes place out of which neuropeptides are produced. At this junction point between the two sides of our being, Ayurveda recognizes three basic governing agents, which are known as *doshas*. The three doshas—which are called Vata, Pitta, and Kapha—can be defined in modern scientific terms, and this definition is our next primary energy principle.

> PEP 7. Vata, Pitta, and Kapha are the fundamental quantum mechanical mind/body mechanisms that govern the flow of intelligence and energy throughout an individual physiology.

There is much to say about each of the doshas, but their basic functions can be defined broadly and simply: Vata dosha is the governing principle in the body that controls movement; Pitta dosha controls metabolism and digestion; and Kapha dosha is responsible for physical structure and fluid balance.

Every cell in your body must contain all three of these principles in order to maintain life. You must have Vata for motion, in order to breathe, to circulate the blood, to move food through the digestive tract, and to send nerve impulses to and from the brain. You must have Pitta in order to assimilate and process food, air, and water through the various systems of your body. You need Kapha, or structure, to hold your cells together and to form muscles, fat, bones, and connective tissue.

Although nature needs all three principles to build and sustain human life, each of us has different proportions of the doshas in our basic constitutions. For example, when I say that a person is a "Vata type," I mean that certain Vata characteristics are dominant in that person's makeup. Pitta types or Kapha types will have their own predominant characteristics.

By identifying and understanding your body type, you can bring your diet, your daily routine, and even your casual behavior into perfect harmony with your physiology as a whole—and you can begin to gain access to your inner reserves of energy. Let's look more closely at the characteristics of the three body types.

VATA

Vata is the governing principle of movement. The influence of Vata in an individual human being can be compared to the action of the wind in nature. Like the wind, Vata is always moving and tends to be quick, cold, dry, rough, and light. People who are Vata types are dominated by these qualities as well.

Characteristics of Vata Type

- Light, thin build
- Performs activity quickly
- Irregular hunger and digestion
- Light, interrupted sleep; tendency toward insomnia
- Enthusiasm, vivaciousness, imagination
- Excitability, changing moods
- Quick to grasp new information, also quick to forget
- Tendency to worry
- Tendency to be constipated
- Tires easily, tendency to overexert
- Mental and physical energy comes in bursts

It is very Vata to

- Be hungry at any time of the day or night
- Love excitement and constant change
- Go to sleep at different times every night, skip meals, and keep irregular habits in general
- Digest food well one day and poorly the next
- Display bursts of emotion that are short-lived and quickly forgotten
- Walk quickly

The basic theme of the Vata type is "changeable." Vata people are unpredictable and much less stereotyped than either Pittas or Kaphas. Their variability—in size, shape, mood, and action—is their defining characteristic. For a Vata person, mental and physical energy comes in bursts. Vata people tend to walk quickly, to be hungry at any hour, to love excitement and change, to go to sleep at a different time every night, to skip meals, and to digest food well one day and poorly the next.

PITTA

Pitta dosha governs digestion and metabolism. Pitta is responsible for all the biochemical transformations that take place in the body, and it is closely involved with hormone and enzyme production. Pitta in the body is likened to the fire principle in nature—it burns, transforms, and digests. Pitta is hot, sharp, and acidic, and Pitta types generally display these qualities.

Characteristics of Pitta Type

- Medium build
- Medium strength and endurance
- Sharp hunger and thirst, strong digestion
- Tendency to become angry or irritable under stress
- Fair or ruddy skin, often freckled
- Aversion to sun, hot weather
- Enterprising character, likes challenges
- Sharp intellect
- Precise, articulate speech
- Cannot skip meals
- Blond, light brown, or red hair (or reddish undertones)

It is very Pitta to

- Feel ravenous if dinner is half an hour late
- Live by your watch and resent having your time wasted
- Wake up at night feeling hot and thirsty
- Take command of a situation or feel that you should
- Learn from experience that others find you too demanding, sarcastic, or critical at times
- Have a determined stride when you walk

Intensity is the theme of the Pitta type. Bright red hair and a florid face indicate a predominance of Pitta, as do ambition, sharp-wittedness, outspokenness, boldness, and a tendency to be argumentative or jealous. But the combative side of Pitta does not have to be blatantly or crudely expressed. When in balance, Pittas are warm, loving, and content. It is very Pitta to walk with a determined stride, to feel ravenously hungry if a meal is half an hour late, to wake up at night feeling thirsty, to live by the clock, and to resent having your time wasted.

KAPHA

Kapha dosha is responsible for structure in the body. In Ayurveda, Kapha is said to be related to the earth and water principles in nature. Kapha dosha is typically heavy, stable, steady, cold, oily, slow, dull, and soft, and Kapha types are characterized by these earthy qualities.

Characteristics of Kapha Type

- Solid, powerful build; great physical strength and endurance
- Steady energy; slow and graceful in action
- Tranquil, relaxed personality; slow to anger
- Cool, smooth, thick, pale, and often oily skin
- Slow to grasp new information, but good retentive memory
- Heavy, prolonged sleep
- Tendency toward obesity
- Slow digestion, mild hunger
- Affectionate, tolerant, forgiving
- Tendency to be possessive, complacent

It is very Kapha to

- Mull things over for a long time before making a decision
- Wake up slowly, lie in bed a long time, and need coffee upon arising
- Be happy with the status quo and preserve it by conciliating others
- Respect other people's feelings (with which you feel genuine empathy)
- Seek emotional comfort from eating
- Have graceful movements, liquid eyes, and a gliding walk, even if overweight

The basic theme of the Kapha type is "relaxed." Kapha dosha brings stability and steadiness, and it provides the physical strength and stamina that define the sturdy frames of typical Kapha people. Kaphas are considered fortunate in Ayurveda because they generally enjoy sound health and a serene, happy view of the world. It is very Kapha to mull things over before making a decision, to sleep soundly and awaken slowly, to seek emotional comfort from food, to be content with the status quo, and to conciliate others in order to preserve it.

DISCOVERING YOUR BODY TYPE

So far our intention has been to introduce the doshas and to show how they can be distinguished from one another. But it's important to understand that most people are "bi-doschic." Their constitutions are structured around a combination of two body types, and in some cases, all three.

The practical effect of these ideas will become clearer when you complete the following questionnaire, which is designed to help you determine your own dosha influences. Before you read any further, I suggest setting aside about thirty minutes for answering the following questions and evaluating your responses.

AYURVEDA BODY-TYPE QUESTIONNAIRE

The following quiz is divided into three sections. For the first 20 questions, which apply to Vata dosha, read each statement and mark, from 0 to 6, whether it applies to you.

0 = Doesn't apply to me
3 = Applies to me somewhat (or some of the time)
6 = Applies to me mostly (or nearly all of the time)

At the end of the section, write down your total Vata score. For example, if you mark a 6 for the first question, a 3 for the second, and a 2 for the third, your total up to that point would be 6 + 3 + 2 = 11. Total the entire section in this way, and you will arrive at your final Vata score. Proceed to the 20 questions for Pitta and those for Kapha.

When you are finished, you will have three separate scores. Comparing these will determine your body type.

For fairly objective physical traits, your choice will usually be obvious. For mental traits and behavior, which are more subjective, you should answer according to how you have felt and acted most of your life, or at least for the past few years.

SECTION 1: VATA

	Does not apply		Applies sometimes			Applies most times	
1. I perform activity very quickly.	0	1	2	3	4	5	6
2. I am not good at memorizing things and then remembering them later.	0	1	2	3	4	5	6
3. I am enthusiastic and vivacious by nature.	0	1	2	3	4	5	6
4. I have a thin physique—I don't gain weight very easily.	0	1	2	3	4	5	6
5. I have always learned new things very quickly.	0	1	2	3	4	5	6
6. My characteristic gait while walking is light and quick.	0	1	2	3	4	5	6
7. I tend to have difficulty making decisions.	0	1	2	3	4	5	6
8. I tend to develop gas and become constipated easily.	0	1	2	3	4	5	6
9. I tend to have cold hands and feet.	0	1	2	3	4	5	6
10. I become anxious or worried frequently.	0	1	2	3	4	5	6

	Does not apply		Applies sometimes			Applies most times
11. I don't tolerate cold weather as well as most people.	0	1	2	3	4	5	6
12. I speak quickly and my friends think that I'm talkative.	0	1	2	3	4	5	6
13. My moods change easily and I am somewhat emotional by nature.	0	1	2	3	4	5	6
14. I often have difficulty falling asleep or having a sound night's sleep.	0	1	2	3	4	5	6
15. My skin tends to be very dry, especially in winter.	0	1	2	3	4	5	6
16. My mind is very active, sometimes restless, but also very imaginative.	0	1	2	3	4	5	6
17. My movements are quick and active; my energy tends to come in bursts.	0	1	2	3	4	5	6
18. I am easily excitable.	0	1	2	3	4	5	6
19. I tend to be irregular in my eating and sleeping habits.	0	1	2	3	4	5	6
20. I learn quickly, but I also forget quickly.	0	1	2	3	4	5	6

VATA SCORE

SECTION 2: PITTA

	Does not apply		Applies sometimes			Applies most times
1. I consider myself to be very efficient.	0	1	2	3	4	5	6
2. In my activities, I tend to be extremely precise and orderly.	0	1	2	3	4	5	6
3. I am strong-minded and have a somewhat forceful manner.	0	1	2	3	4	5	6
4. I feel uncomfortable or become easily fatigued in hot weather—more so than other people.	0	1	2	3	4	5	6
5. I tend to perspire easily.	0	1	2	3	4	5	6
6. Even though I might not always show it, I become irritable or angry quite easily.	0	1	2	3	4	5	6

	Does not apply		Applies sometimes			Applies most times
7. If I skip a meal or a meal is delayed, I become uncomfortable.	0	1	2	3	4	5	6
8. One or more of the following characteristics describes my hair: • early graying or balding • thin, fine, straight • blond, red, or sandy-colored	0	1	2	3	4	5	6
9. I have a strong appetite; if I want to, I can eat quite a large quantity.	0	1	2	3	4	5	6
10. Many people consider me stubborn.	0	1	2	3	4	5	6
11. I am very regular in my bowel habits—it would be more common for me to have loose stools than to be constipated.	0	1	2	3	4	5	6
12. I become impatient very easily.	0	1	2	3	4	5	6
13. I tend to be a perfectionist about details.	0	1	2	3	4	5	6
14. I get angry quite easily, but then I quickly forget about it.	0	1	2	3	4	5	6
15. I am very fond of cold foods, such as ice cream, and also ice-cold drinks.	0	1	2	3	4	5	6
16. I am more likely to feel that a room is too hot than too cold.	0	1	2	3	4	5	6
17. I don't tolerate foods that are very hot and spicy.	0	1	2	3	4	5	6
18. I am not as tolerant of disagreement as I should be.	0	1	2	3	4	5	6
19. I enjoy challenges, and when I want something I am very determined in my efforts to get it.	0	1	2	3	4	5	6
20. I tend to be quite critical of others and also of myself.	0	1	2	3	4	5	6

PITTA SCORE

SECTION 3: KAPHA

	Does not apply			Applies sometimes			Applies most times
1. My natural tendency is to do things in a slow and relaxed fashion.	0	1	2	3	4	5	6
2. I gain weight more easily than most people and lose it more slowly.	0	1	2	3	4	5	6
3. I have a placid and calm disposition—I'm not easily ruffled.	0	1	2	3	4	5	6
4. I can skip meals easily without any significant discomfort.	0	1	2	3	4	5	6
5. I have a tendency toward excess mucus or phlegm, chronic congestion asthma, or sinus problems.	0	1	2	3	4	5	6
6. I must get at least eight hours of sleep in order to be comfortable the next day.	0	1	2	3	4	5	6
7. I sleep very deeply.	0	1	2	3	4	5	6
8. I am calm by nature and not easily angered.	0	1	2	3	4	5	6
9. I don't learn as quickly as some people, but I have excellent retention and a long memory.	0	1	2	3	4	5	6
10. I have a tendency toward becoming plump—I store extra fat easily.	0	1	2	3	4	5	6
11. Weather that is cool and damp bothers me.	0	1	2	3	4	5	6
12. My hair is thick, dark, and wavy.	0	1	2	3	4	5	6
13. I have smooth, soft skin with a somewhat pale complexion.	0	1	2	3	4	5	6
14. I have a large, solid body build.	0	1	2	3	4	5	6
15. The following words describe me well: serene, sweet-natured, affectionate, and forgiving.	0	1	2	3	4	5	6
16. I have slow digestion, which makes me feel heavy after eating.	0	1	2	3	4	5	6
17. I have very good stamina and physical endurance as well as a steady level of energy.	0	1	2	3	4	5	6

	Does not apply		Applies sometimes			Applies most times	
18. I generally walk with a slow, measured gait.	0	1	2	3	4	5	6
19. I have a tendency toward oversleeping, and grogginess upon awakening, and am generally slow to get going in the morning.	0	1	2	3	4	5	6
20. I am a slow eater and am slow and methodical in my actions.	0	1	2	3	4	5	6

KAPHA SCORE

FINAL SCORE

VATA PITTA KAPHA

HOW TO DETERMINE YOUR BODY TYPE

Now that you have added up your scores, you can determine your body type. Although there are only three doshas, remember that Ayurveda combines them in ten ways to arrive at ten different body types.

- **If one score is much higher than the others, you are probably a single-dosha type.**

  Single-Dosha Types
  Vata
  Pitta
  Kapha

You are definitely a single-dosha type if one score is twice as high as another dosha score (for instance, Vata—90, Pitta—45, Kapha—35), but a smaller margin also applies. In single-dosha types, the characteristics of Vata, Pitta, or Kapha predominate. Your next highest dosha will still show up in your natural tendencies, but it will be much less distinct.

- **If no single dosha dominates, you are a two-dosha type.**

  Two-Dosha Types
  Vata-Pitta or Pitta-Vata
  Pitta-Kapha or Kapha-Pitta
  Vata-Kapha or Kapha-Vata

If you are a two-dosha type, the traits of your two leading doshas will predominate. The higher one comes first in your body type, but both count.

Most people are two-dosha types. A two-dosha type might have a score like this: Vata—80, Pitta—90, Kapha—20. If this was your score, you would consider yourself to be a Pitta-Vata type.

- **If your three scores are nearly equal, you may be a three-dosha type.**

  Three-Dosha Type
  Vata-Pitta-Kapha

However, this type is considered rarest of all. Check your answers again, or have a friend go over your responses with you. Also, you can read over the descriptions of Vata, Pitta, and Kapha on pages 16–20 to see if one or two doshas are more prominent in your makeup.

Now that you have an idea of your particular constitutional type, take a moment to review the qualities of the doshas in order to learn which are most influential in your physiology. This information will be most helpful as you begin using the practical techniques that will be presented in subsequent chapters.

The key point to remember is that, according to the Ayurvedic mind/body system, optimum physical and mental health derives from proper balance of the doshas. When the basic governing principles of mind and body are coordinated, perfect harmony exists between the physical and spiritual sides of our nature. Energy, vitality, and overall good health are the natural result.

PEP 8. Balance of the doshas brings about coordination of the entire mind/body physiology. When the doshas are balanced, all of the body's systems work together to create energy, strength, and health.

Although *balance* is a key word, it expresses itself differently in different individuals. A balanced Vata person, for example, will display characteristics that are distinctly different from those of a balanced Kapha person. Moreover, these two body types require different influences in order to remain in balance. Vata types, who are naturally light and airy, need to create more heaviness and stability in the mind/body system; these "airy" types need more "earthy" influences. In contrast, Kapha types need to "lighten up" in order to remain balanced; they should seek out influences that get them into action both mentally and physically. Starting right now, try to use what you've learned about your body type to help you make better choices in all areas of your life, including your diet, exercise, sleep schedule, and even in your work and personal relationships.

DOSHA IMBALANCES

When a dosha goes out of balance, it no longer exists in the correct proportion required by an individual's body type. One influence has become so active that it dominates or eclipses the other mind/body qualities. The natural condition of harmony in the physiology, prakriti, has been replaced by the state of imbalance called *vikriti*. This can be the basis for many health concerns, including chronic fatigue.

In general, fatigue is most often a problem of Vata-type individuals. Their energy tends to come in sudden, powerful bursts, but their stamina is often weak. At a given moment they may feel so exhilarated that they push themselves beyond their natural limits. While they are enthusiastic and vivacious by nature, pure Vata types are also most likely to feel the stresses of a demanding schedule or a busy lifestyle. Though they may seem to thrive on overactivity for a time, they eventually become emotionally drained and physically exhausted. Of the three basic body types, Vatas must be most careful about monitoring their energy resources and using them in a balanced way.

Chronic fatigue can also afflict individuals who are predominantly Pitta or Kapha, but there is usually a more specific and clearly identifiable reason for their tiredness. Pitta fatigue may be caused by situations that overheat or "inflame" the Pitta nature, such as excessive sunlight, hot or acidic foods, or emotions such as anger, envy, and irritability. One of the most common causes of chronic fatigue in Pitta types is a tendency toward overwork. Pittas usually have drive and ambition, but the demands they impose on themselves can outstrip even their naturally abundant energy resources.

The inherent stamina of Kapha types would seem to protect them from chronic fatigue, but Kaphas also tend to accumulate "heaviness," both physically and emotionally. When they go out of balance, they gain weight or experience illnesses such as severe colds or flu, which are associated with fluid congestion and irritated mucous membranes. Dullness and lethargy can come to dominate their personalities. These Kapha symptoms demand a very different response than would be called for by Vata or Pitta imbalance. Chronically fatigued Kaphas need to be up and about. They need influences that demand increased activity. Kaphas should motivate themselves to think sharply and accurately, and they should get their bodies involved in purposeful action.

Here is a summary of fatigue-causing imbalances in each of the three doshas.

• **Vata imbalance** is the most common type of fatigue. It often comes and goes suddenly, but even if it is consistently present it tends to vary in intensity at different times of the day. These sudden changes can be brought about by any sort of major or minor influence—a piece of good news can cause an abrupt infusion of energy, but a stressful situation can result in a sense of exhaustion. Though Vata-type fatigue may be experienced as an overwhelming sensation, everything about Vata is actually light by nature; the individual is usually able to get through daily activities despite feeling tired. Vata fatigue is often accompanied by other Vata symptoms, such as anxiety, insomnia, and low-grade depression.

- **Pitta imbalance** and resulting fatigue is usually associated with overwork, excessive heat, or eating inappropriate foods. Pitta fatigue may be accompanied by perspiration, acid indigestion, and other Pitta symptoms. The most common emotional symptoms accompanying Pitta fatigue are irritability and anger.
- **Kapha imbalance** has a characteristically heavy feeling to it. The tiredness experienced by a Kapha type may seem so profound that even slight movements seem difficult, and there can be an overwhelming sense of inertia. Kapha fatigue is often associated with accumulations of impurities or toxins in the system, which can literally "dampen" the energy producing mechanisms of the body. Kapha fatigue may also be related to severe emotional depression.

THE POWER OF ATTENTION

Below is another Primary Energy Principle that should be extremely helpful as you continue to use the Energy Tracking Chart at the end of chapter 1. Remember that the Energy Tracking Chart will help you get in touch with your hidden energy resources. Please continue to use it three times a day as new techniques are introduced in subsequent chapters.

As with all the PEPs, I suggest you write this one down, too:

PEP 9. Whatever we put our attention on grows stronger in our lives. The quality of our attention determines whether benefit or harm results.

Attention is the projection of energy and consciousness, and it is a powerful force. Whatever we put our attention on tends to increase, for good or for ill. Properly directed attention can have a nourishing quality; it can be a beam of positive awareness that heals body and mind. But negative attention can exacerbate any physical or mental symptom.

If there is some imbalance present in your mind/body system, nature will direct your attention toward it through signals of discomfort or pain. At that point, you have a choice to make regarding the positive or negative quality of your awareness. By focusing attention on the debilitating effects of fatigue, you can cause those effects to grow. However, if you make your attention a force for energy and vitality, you can help those qualities to gain strength and promote healing.

It is extremely important to realize that no matter how deep your sense of fatigue may be, there is always a spark of energy alive in your body. The very fact that you're alive and reading this book is an expression of the vital energy that's alive in every part of your mind/body system. By focusing your awareness on that energy, you can turn even a small spark into a bright flame.

3

The Importance of Good Digestion

Everything you do and accomplish every day—from the beating of your heart, to the millions of microscopic processes happening in every one of our cells, to walking and thinking and working—everything requires energy, and it is derived from the food you eat. But where does the energy in the food itself come from? Ultimately, of course, it comes from the sun, which provides the light and the heat that plants need in order to grow. It is through food, therefore, that we as human beings gain access to the energy of the universe.

During digestion, complex molecules of food are broken down into progressively simpler forms. This transformation is called metabolism. Most of the energy from the metabolism of food becomes available during the final stages, when oxygen combines with basic molecules such as simple sugars. This is called oxidation, and it is constantly taking place at lightning speed. The oxygen that you take into your lungs is carried by your blood to every cell of your body. Entering these cells, it combines with food molecules, which have also been brought to the cells in the bloodstream. This mixing of oxygen with simple food molecules is similar to the consumption of fuel in a fireplace, in which large amounts of energy are released from burning wood in the form of heat and light. In a human body, however, energy from the oxidation of food is released in a much more controlled way. As a result, the body is able to capture this energy and store it for future use. It is this energy that enables us to live and to act.

Ayurveda speaks of "digestive fire" as the medium through which energy is released. *Agni,* which means "fire" in Sanskrit, breaks down the food we eat and assimilates it into the system. This digestive fire can be understood as a metaphor for the enzymes that are described by modern physiology.

The production of metabolic energy depends on a number of critical factors, including the kinds of foods you eat, your overall state of health, the amount and quality of the air you breathe, and even the thoughts and emotions you're constantly experiencing.

Much has been written in recent years about the importance of good eating habits to health and vitality. But from an Ayurvedic viewpoint, strength of digestion is even more important than nutrition. Indeed, the nutritional value of any food is only useful to the extent that your body can access it through the digestive process. If digestion is weak, food will not be adequately metabolized and its energy will simply be lost. For this reason, building the power of digestion will be our most important consideration in this chapter.

WEAK DIGESTION AND THE CREATION OF AMA

In addition to the waste of energy and nutritional value, there is another important effect of incomplete digestion. Poor digestion causes a residue of food to accumulate in the body. If not properly eliminated, this residue becomes the basis for a wide variety of impurities and toxins. The Sanskrit word for these residual impurities is *ama*. According to Ayurveda, ama is an extremely significant cause of fatigue and other long-term health problems. In fact, I believe that digestive imbalance and the resulting accumulation of ama is present in virtually every person who suffers from chronic fatigue.

Ayurveda describes ama as a sticky substance that blocks normal channels of flow in the physiology. These include not only the veins and arteries of the circulatory system, but also the ducts that transport all the enzymes and metabolic substances of the body. Because it blocks the normal flow of biological energy, ama is fundamental to the problem of chronic fatigue. It's like a wet blanket that literally smothers the energy-producing fires of the body.

Ama can sometimes be seen in the form of a white coating on the tongue, especially just after awakening. This is because impurities from incomplete digestion come up from the digestive tract during the night and collect in the mouth. Other symptoms of ama are feelings of weakness or heaviness, lethargy, poor immunity, irregular bowl movements, and sharp fluctuations in appetite levels. Of course, chronic fatigue itself is an important sign of ama production.

TECHNIQUES FOR STRENGTHENING DIGESTION

The benefits of strong digestion should be quite clear. It ensures proper assimilation of food and it prevents the accumulation of toxic impurities in the body.

The elements of strong digestion are summarized in our next Primary Energy Principle:

PEP 10. The quality of digestion is a major factor in promoting vital biological energy. The four main factors that affect digestion are: quality of awareness, timing, quantity of food, and quality of food.

Below are some extremely important techniques you can use to strengthen your digestion. These techniques can benefit all three body types, but they will be especially applicable to Vatas, who tend to have irregular digestion, and to Kaphas, whose digestion is often slow.

Implementing these principles may require some changes in your current habits, but the positive effects will be immediately apparent and worthwhile as you move toward a more natural way of eating and digesting.

1. *Eat in a quiet and settled atmosphere.* Don't divide your attention by working, reading, listening to the radio or watching television during mealtimes. If your attention is entirely on your food and its various flavors, your power of digestion will be greatly enhanced. Always remember that awareness has organizing power. When you eat with calm but focused awareness, your digestive fire will be balanced and strong. But if your awareness is distracted, the power of digestion will weaken.
2. *Establish regular mealtimes.* When you eat at the same time every day, your system becomes accustomed to digesting according to that routine, and digestion occurs automatically and thoroughly. Irregular mealtimes "confuse" the mind/body system and disallow thorough digestion. Though many people with busy lifestyles can benefit from this point, Vata types especially can benefit because of their irregular tendencies.
3. *Always sit down to eat.* Even if you're just having a snack, take the time to sit down at the table. This will make your

digestion more thorough, by helping to direct your awareness toward your food.

4. *Don't eat when you're upset.* Eating when you're disturbed or angry divides your awareness. This will definitely weaken the digestive fire and produce ama. If you're under stress, wait a few minutes until you feel more settled. It's also best to avoid any controversial discussions at mealtimes that might cause tension or irritability.
5. *Eat only to a point of comfortable satisfaction.* The quantity of food eaten at each sitting is a very important factor in good digestion. Ayurveda teaches that we should eat to three-fourths of capacity. Eating beyond this point is like smothering a fire with too much fuel. When the stomach is completely full, food is incompletely metabolized because the digestive fire doesn't have enough room to do its work. So stop eating when you feel satisfied, but before you feel heavy and completely full. This will leave some space in your system for digestive enzymes to function effectively.
6. *Avoid ice-cold foods and drinks.* Cold substances tend to freeze the digestive fires. Because Vata and Kapha are both cold by nature, these two doshas will be especially affected by cold foods. Unfortunately, the practice of drinking cold beverages with meals is deeply established in many Americans. You may think this will be a difficult habit to break. But after a week or two most people no longer miss cold drinks and feel much healthier without them.
7. *Don't talk while chewing your food.* While you're eating, your senses should be turned inward in order to enjoy the taste, sight, and aroma of the meal. Make it a rule not to speak while you have food in your mouth. And as previously mentioned, conversations at the table should be calm and light, not emotional or disruptive.

8. *Eat at a moderate pace.* Gulping food makes good digestion difficult, so take enough time to eat your meals slowly. A hurried and harried meal is one of the worst things you can do to your energy and good health. You may think that you'll increase your productivity by eating quickly, but don't be misled—the time you gain in your schedule will be more than offset by increased fatigue. So give mealtimes the respect they deserve. After all, this is the point in the day when vital energy is created, and eating hurriedly is like weakening a tree at its root. Try to regulate the speed with which you eat by not placing the next bite of food on your fork until you have chewed and swallowed the previous bite.
9. *Don't eat anything until your last meal has been completely digested.* Snacking while you're still digesting an earlier meal will produce ama. An analogy can be made with cooking bean soup—if you keep adding beans while the soup is cooking, it will never be done. Digestion of a meal usually takes three to six hours. Hunger is nature's sign that digestion has been completed, so if you're not feeling hungry, don't eat. If you don't seem to be hungry at mealtimes (and you haven't been snacking) it may be that accumulated ama is dulling your appetite. In such a case, you should eat moderately to avoid overwhelming the digestive fire and producing still more ama. If you feel ravenously hungry between meals and absolutely must have a snack, make it something light, such as a piece of fruit.
10. *Sit quietly for a few minutes after your meal.* This allows digestion to begin effortlessly. If possible, it's even better to lie down for fifteen or twenty minutes.

Let me emphasize once more that the small effort required by these techniques will be greatly rewarded. If you've grown attached to certain unhealthy patterns—watching TV while eating, for example—remind yourself that it is these same habits that weaken your digestion, produce ama, and contribute to chronic fatigue.

It's not necessary to implement all ten techniques at once. Start with the ones that seem easiest to you. The checklist that follows on pages 38–39 can help you incorporate these new behaviors into your daily routine: once you've grown accustomed to the easier techniques, add a new one each week until you've got them all. This will also allow you to monitor your energy levels as new techniques are put into practice.

ADDITIONAL TECHNIQUES

The ideas we've discussed so far involve only behaviors at mealtimes. Here are three more Ayurvedic practices for improving digestion and eliminating ama from the system. I am going to discuss these separately from the other techniques because they're somewhat more sophisticated and may require a bit more of a lifestyle adjustment. However, most people find these ideas are of great benefit to digestion and to energizing the entire body/mind system.

These methods work by preventing the production of ama or by thoroughly cleansing it from the system. Here is the Primary Energy Principle that is the foundation of these techniques:

> PEP 11. Incomplete or imbalanced digestion gives rise to physiological impurities called ama that block the free flow of energy in the body. Vital energy is enhanced by preventing the accumulation of these impurities and cleansing them from the system.

The first new principle is to *eat your main meal of the day at lunchtime rather than in the evening.* Our contemporary habit

BODY INTELLIGENCE TECHNIQUES CHECKLIST

Start using your checklist every time you eat, whether it is a full meal or a snack. This will help you monitor your progress in applying the techniques. If some of them seem too difficult, try the easy ones first. Then add a new technique every week until you have incorporated them all. For the first meal of the day, use the circles numbered with a 1 to check off the techniques you used. If you did not use a Body Intelligence Technique, leave the space blank. There are enough spaces to record four meals or snacks a day.

	Monday	Tuesday	Wednesday	Thursday	Friday	Saturday	Sunday
Ate in a settled and quiet atmosphere	1○ 2○ 3○ 4○	1○ 2○ 3○ 4○	1○ 2○ 3○ 4○	1○ 2○ 3○ 4○	1○ 2○ 3○ 4○	1○ 2○ 3○ 4○	1○ 2○ 3○ 4○
Ate at my regularly scheduled mealtime	1○ 2○ 3○ 4○	1○ 2○ 3○ 4○	1○ 2○ 3○ 4○	1○ 2○ 3○ 4○	1○ 2○ 3○ 4○	1○ 2○ 3○ 4○	1○ 2○ 3○ 4○
Sat down at a table to eat	1○ 2○ 3○ 4○	1○ 2○ 3○ 4○	1○ 2○ 3○ 4○	1○ 2○ 3○ 4○	1○ 2○ 3○ 4○	1○ 2○ 3○ 4○	1○ 2○ 3○ 4○
Didn't eat when upset	1○ 2○ 3○ 4○	1○ 2○ 3○ 4○	1○ 2○ 3○ 4○	1○ 2○ 3○ 4○	1○ 2○ 3○ 4○	1○ 2○ 3○ 4○	1○ 2○ 3○ 4○
Stopped eating when only 3/4 full	1○ 2○ 3○ 4○	1○ 2○ 3○ 4○	1○ 2○ 3○ 4○	1○ 2○ 3○ 4○	1○ 2○ 3○ 4○	1○ 2○ 3○ 4○	1○ 2○ 3○ 4○

Avoided cold foods and drinks	1 ○ 2 ○ 3 ○ 4 ○	1 ○ 2 ○ 3 ○ 4 ○	1 ○ 2 ○ 3 ○ 4 ○	1 ○ 2 ○ 3 ○ 4 ○	1 ○ 2 ○ 3 ○ 4 ○	1 ○ 2 ○ 3 ○ 4 ○	1 ○ 2 ○ 3 ○ 4 ○
Didn't talk while chewing	1 ○ 2 ○ 3 ○ 4 ○	1 ○ 2 ○ 3 ○ 4 ○	1 ○ 2 ○ 3 ○ 4 ○	1 ○ 2 ○ 3 ○ 4 ○	1 ○ 2 ○ 3 ○ 4 ○	1 ○ 2 ○ 3 ○ 4 ○	1 ○ 2 ○ 3 ○ 4 ○
Ate at a moderate pace	1 ○ 2 ○ 3 ○ 4 ○	1 ○ 2 ○ 3 ○ 4 ○	1 ○ 2 ○ 3 ○ 4 ○	1 ○ 2 ○ 3 ○ 4 ○	1 ○ 2 ○ 3 ○ 4 ○	1 ○ 2 ○ 3 ○ 4 ○	1 ○ 2 ○ 3 ○ 4 ○
Ate only after the previous meal had been completely digested	1 ○ 2 ○ 3 ○ 4 ○	1 ○ 2 ○ 3 ○ 4 ○	1 ○ 2 ○ 3 ○ 4 ○	1 ○ 2 ○ 3 ○ 4 ○	1 ○ 2 ○ 3 ○ 4 ○	1 ○ 2 ○ 3 ○ 4 ○	1 ○ 2 ○ 3 ○ 4 ○
Ate a freshly cooked and balanced meal	1 ○ 2 ○ 3 ○ 4 ○	1 ○ 2 ○ 3 ○ 4 ○	1 ○ 2 ○ 3 ○ 4 ○	1 ○ 2 ○ 3 ○ 4 ○	1 ○ 2 ○ 3 ○ 4 ○	1 ○ 2 ○ 3 ○ 4 ○	1 ○ 2 ○ 3 ○ 4 ○
Sat quietly for a few minutes after eating	1 ○ 2 ○ 3 ○ 4 ○	1 ○ 2 ○ 3 ○ 4 ○	1 ○ 2 ○ 3 ○ 4 ○	1 ○ 2 ○ 3 ○ 4 ○	1 ○ 2 ○ 3 ○ 4 ○	1 ○ 2 ○ 3 ○ 4 ○	1 ○ 2 ○ 3 ○ 4 ○

of eating a large meal around 6:00 P.M. may be one of our biggest diet-related mistakes, and it is a major cause of chronic fatigue.

Our internal biological rhythms are connected to the rhythms of the natural world around us. Therefore the internal digestive fire is brightest at the same time that the sun is highest in the sky, and according to Ayurveda, digestion is sharpest at noontime. If you eat a large quantity of food at this time, it will be thoroughly digested and assimilated and you'll get energy without producing ama. But this will not be the case if the same volume of food is consumed at a later hour.

Similarly, the Western custom of eating a large breakfast may also be detrimental to health and energy. Digestion is sluggish in the early morning just after you've awakened. Therefore Ayurveda recommends a light meal early in the day, like the European continental breakfast. In fact, if you aren't very hungry in the morning it's perfectly reasonable to skip breakfast altogether and save the digestive fire for use at lunch.

Because most of us are accustomed to a large meal in the evening, it may be a challenge to put this recommendation into effect immediately. Also, work and other scheduling considerations can make lunchtime a quick affair for many and a nonevent for some. But try to become aware of the major toll that such habits inflict on your body. By really devoting some attention to it, almost anyone can find a creative way to have a more substantial lunch, even if it means preparing the meal the night before. Or it may simply involve locating a good restaurant near your place of work. If this still seems difficult for you, start with one or two days each week and see how you feel. And remember that breakfast and your evening meal should be relatively light.

My second recommendation is a purification technique for removing ama from the system. It's very straightforward, but it's also very profound and effective. All you're asked to do is *sip hot water frequently throughout the day, as often as every half-hour.* Many people with chronic fatigue, as well as other long-term health problems, have found that this technique alone can greatly benefit the problem.

Get a good quality thermos and fill it with freshly boiled water each morning. Bring the water to a strong boil, then reduce the flame and allow it to heat more slowly for five to ten minutes. This gives the water more energy and makes it a more effective purifier. When you've filled your thermos, keep it with you all day and sip from it frequently. It may help to put the thermos where you can see it easily as a reminder.

You should take one or two sips of hot water every half-hour throughout the day. If you're thirsty, of course, you should feel free to drink more than a few sips at a time. The constant exposure to the cleansing influence of the water will eliminate ama from your body, while the warmth will help to dilate and relax your intestines and allow for a good flushing of the system. Please note that this technique is fundamentally different from weight-control plans that stipulate consumption of large amounts of water every day. It is not the quantity of water that is emphasized here; it is the frequency and the temperature, which are important in creating the purifying effect.

If you find it impossible to sip water as often as every half-hour, just do the best you can. Many people ask if anything can be added to hot water to make it more interesting. Although plain water is the best cleanser, once or twice a day you can add some lemon, which can even have an additional cleansing effect. You shouldn't drink lemon water every half-hour, however.

The third new technique for improving digestion and eliminating ama is to *periodically take a full day during which you consume only liquids and eat no solid foods.* This allows your gastrointestinal organs to take a twenty-four-hour rest. Impurities will be cleansed from your system during that interval, and afterward your digestive fire will be rekindled, stronger than before.

Feel free to consume anything you want as long as it's in liquid form. This includes hot water, fresh fruit juices or vegetable juices, broths, or herbal teas. I especially recommend a yogurt drink, which Ayurveda calls *lassi,* which can be made in both sweet and salty varieties. Here are recipes for two varieties of lassi.

- **Sweet Lassi.** Mix ¼ to ½ cup of yogurt with ½ cup of room temperature water in a blender. Add a pinch of cardamom and honey to taste. Blend thoroughly. Makes one serving.
- **Sour Lassi.** Same as above, but omit cardamom and honey while substituting a pinch of ground cumin and a pinch of salt to taste. Blend thoroughly.

The frequency with which you undertake the one-day liquid diet should be determined by your body type. For Kaphas, the liquid diet should take place one day out of every seven. It's best to pick the same day each week, and it should be a day when you're not likely to have many responsibilities, such as Sunday. Pitta types, who tend to have stronger hunger, should use the liquid diet about once every two weeks, while Vata types should use it only about once a month. This is because Vatas may become weak and uncomfortable without solid food, even for one day. They need some "earthy" property each day to promote balance.

If you are a Vata or a Pitta type, and you find that the liquid diet is making you uncomfortable, try including boiled milk or lassi. If you still experience discomfort, modify the procedure by eating a light but solid evening meal instead of remaining on only liquids until bedtime. Occasionally, even with this alteration, some people find the liquid diet too difficult to follow without encountering problems. If this is your experience, just skip this technique entirely.

If you can gradually incorporate all the methods presented

in this chapter for preserving and strengthening digestion, you will soon notice dramatic improvement in your energy levels. Use the Body Intelligence Techniques Checklist in this chapter to help make the techniques part of your everyday routine. Remember to start with the ideas that seem easiest for you, and then add a new one each week. But try to implement the last three recommendations—lunch as the major meal, the thermos of hot water, and the liquid diet—as soon as possible. Many people notice rapid benefits from these. The benefits should be made apparent as you continue to use the Energy Tracking Chart in chapter 1 throughout the day.

Having considered the importance of good digestion in eliminating fatigue, we're now ready to discuss the various foods that should be emphasized and avoided. There's no doubt that certain foods are natural energizers while others are inherently fatigue-producing. We'll consider this important topic in the next chapter.

4

Diet and Energy

Although the quality of your digestion is of primary importance for creating healthy levels of energy, the selection of foods you eat every day is also extremely significant for combatting fatigue and maintaining overall health. This is the subject of our first diet-related Primary Energy Principle. Please write it in your notes:

> PEP 12. Certain foods are natural energizers, while others can dull the body and the mind, and produce fatigue. The effect of a given food depends on its inherent qualities, as well as how it was obtained, prepared, and consumed.

Think for a moment about the kinds of foods you've eaten during the past few days. Did these include leftovers or fast foods? If so, you've been sacrificing energy and health for the sake of convenience, and you've been denying important nutritional benefits to your body. This is because leftover or highly processed foods lack freshness and, according to Ayurveda, lack vital energy as well. They are so removed from the sources of vitality in nature that they often do little more than create lethargy and inertia. And because such foods are more difficult to digest, they easily lead to the formation of ama.

Once a food has been cooked, you should make every effort to eat it within four or five hours at most. After that time, any food tends to become dull and inert. Our contemporary practice of cooking food, eating some of it, refrigerating the rest, and then warming it again later is neither natural nor healthy from an Ayurvedic perspective. Of course, it's difficult to avoid leftovers if your lifestyle really depends on them, but I strongly urge you to reduce any dependence on reheated meals and to increase the proportion of freshly prepared food in your diet. Frozen foods are also less than ideal, although they occupy a slightly different category than leftovers. Supermarket vegetables that have been frozen raw, for example, have much more vital energy than reheated vegetables. But the best foods are those that are freshest. Although all fresh foods have an energizing effect, it's especially beneficial to include fresh fruit and freshly squeezed juices in your diet. Carrot juice and beet juice are particularly good energizers.

ENERGY-PRODUCING FOODS

In Ayurveda, there is a word that describes naturally energizing foods; they are called *sattvic*. Foods that produce dullness and inertia are called *tamasic*. Foods that are considered especially rich in natural energy, and are therefore especially useful for alleviating fatigue, include the following:

- Fresh fruits and vegetables
- Whole milk, or ghee (clarified butter)

- Wheat and wheat products, including breads and pastas
- Rice, barley, and honey
- Raisins, dates, figs, and almonds
- Olive oil
- Mung beans, and especially mung soup, which is called *dhal* in Ayurveda

These are by no means the only foods that create energy, and you will almost certainly want to include others in your diet. It is worth noting, however, that a complete and nutritious diet—a sattvic diet—can be constructed solely from the foods on this list.

Vegetables

Although Ayurveda definitely advocates eating fresh fruits and vegetables, "fresh" does not mean "raw." I recommend cooking vegetables because cooking improves their digestibility. Raw vegetables are relatively hard for the body to process, so their vitamins and minerals are unlikely to be properly assimilated. But if you do like to eat raw vegetables, the best time to do so is at the beginning of lunch, when the digestive fire is at its highest. Eating a raw salad with lunch will also provide dietary fiber and help tone the whole digestive tract. At other times during the day cooked vegetables are best.

Vegetables that grow above the earth and are completely exposed to sunlight are considered more energizing than those growing below the ground. Two exceptions to this rule are carrots and beets, which are considered very good energizers. Other beneficial vegetables include all the green leafy varieties, fresh herbs such as parsley and basil, and mung bean sprouts. I particularly recommend favoring such vegetables in your lunchtime salad, and in cooked form at other times of the day.

Dairy Products

Ayurveda teaches that milk should be boiled in order to make it more easily digestible. Drinking cold milk can produce a variety of problems, including mucous congestion, diarrhea, and other symptoms that are commonly called "milk allergy." Milk is a very sattvic food, however, and can provide excellent energy value. Try adding a few pinches of fresh grated ginger to your milk before boiling. Or you can use two pinches of turmeric spice, and then, after it's cooled a bit, sweeten the milk with a little honey or sugar.

There's no doubt that improving your digestion of milk can provide access to a new source of energy and stamina. Try to get the freshest dairy products available. Ayurveda recommends whole milk unless you have high cholesterol. Check with your doctor if you're unsure about your cholesterol level.

Ghee is clarified butter, which means that the butter has been purified by heating. It is considered in Ayurveda to be an extremely energizing substance. You can use ghee instead of butter on toast or other foods, and it also makes an excellent cooking oil because it does not burn. A small to moderate amount of ghee in your diet will help improve your absorption and assimilation of food. If cholesterol is a problem, you should avoid ghee or use it only in very small amounts.

Ghee can be purchased in health food stores and in many groceries. Or you can make it yourself, using the following recipe:

HOW TO PREPARE GHEE

1. In a deep stainless steel pan, place one or more pounds of unsalted butter over medium-to-low heat. Watch closely that the butter doesn't scorch while melting.
2. As the butter heats, its water content will boil away. Af-

ter thirty to forty minutes, milk solids will appear on the surface of the liquid and at the bottom of the pan.

3. As the milk solids turn golden brown at the bottom of the pan, remove the liquid ghee from the heat. Be careful that the ghee doesn't burn. The ghee may smell like popcorn at this point, and you might notice tiny bubbles rising from the bottom.
4. Cover a stainless steel strainer with a cotton cloth, and pour the ghee through it while it's still hot. Use a stainless steel or glass bowl to catch the ghee as it pours through the strainer.
5. It is not necessary to refrigerate ghee, but you may if you wish.

Yogurt

Yogurt can also be an energizing food, but freshness is extremely important. Since it becomes increasingly tamasic and ama-producing as it sits on the shelf, the best yogurt is that which you make yourself at home. This is much simpler than it sounds. Yogurt makers are available in many stores and it takes only about five minutes in the evening to make a batch of yogurt that will be fresh for eating the next day. Here is the procedure:

How to Make Yogurt

1. Purchase an electric yogurt maker that maintains a constant temperature. Choose one that has several small cups rather than a single large container, and be sure it includes a thermometer. Then buy whole cow's milk from the grocery store to use as a starter.
2. Measure one cup of milk for every 3/4 cup of yogurt that you plan to use the following day. Pour the milk into a stainless steel pan, and boil it briefly. You can add a few slices of fresh ginger to make the milk more digestible.

3. Using a thermometer, let the milk cool to between 106 and 110 degrees. Then pour the milk into the cups of the yogurt maker, and add about 1/4 tablespoon of yogurt to each cup. Do not stir.
4. Plug in the yogurt maker. It usually takes about nine hours for the yogurt to set. Follow the directions that come with your yogurt maker.
5. Each day, save part of your yogurt as a starter for your next batch. Plan to make fresh yogurt daily. The best time to start is around 9:00 P.M., so the yogurt can sit overnight and be ready the next morning.

Herbs

In Ayurveda, certain herbs are known to have unique energizing and revitalizing properties. These herbs are combined according to specific traditional formulas to create compounds known as *rasayanas*. Knowledge of rasayanas is an ancient part of the Ayurvedic mind/body system, and they are described in detail in the classical texts. Rasayana compounds were used by the ancient kings and *rishis* (sages) of India to promote long life and vitality.

Much knowledge of rasayanas became lost or misunderstood during the centuries when India was occupied by foreign governments. During this period Ayurveda was actively suppressed. Now, however, formulas for some of the most important classical rasayanas have been restored, and these preparations are now being created according to the traditional recipes. The most important of these compounds is called Amrit Kalash. It comes in two forms: an herbal paste, called Nectar, and an herbal tablet, called Ambrosia. Both of these preparations have a strengthening and balancing effect on the entire system. I recommend that you consider taking these rasayanas as an optional but valuable supplement to the other ideas and techniques presented here. Information on obtaining rasayanas can be found in the sources at the end of this book.

ENERGY-DEPLETING FOODS

Foods that reduce energy—tamasic foods—may be difficult to digest, or they may contain some inherently fatigue-producing toxins. Ayurveda considers the foods below to have an energy-depleting effect:

- Red meat, including beef, pork, and veal
- Aged or fermented foods, including aged or sour cheeses, and pickled or smoked foods
- Onions, garlic, and mushrooms
- Potatoes and other vegetables that grow below the ground. Carrots and beets are exceptions.
- Refined sugar, alcohol, and coffee

Red Meat and Other Meat Products

It's significant that the first item on the tamasic food list is red meat. Because fruits and vegetables are considered to be purer and more energizing than animal foods, Ayurveda teaches that diet should come from vegetarian food sources. These sources provide greater vitality for a very simple reason: they are lower on the food chain and closer to the sun, which is the original source of energy in food.

There is considerable loss of energy when vegetable foods are consumed by animals and converted into meat. In simple grains, for example, energy value is about seven times more concentrated than in meat from the animals who ate those grains. So if you want to feed a hog enough to create one unit of pork for human consumption, you must use seven units of grain to create that one unit of pork. Researchers have estimated that if the American public—who are the largest consumers of meat in the world—were to reduce their consumption of meat by even 10 percent, this would liberate sufficient resources of grain to feed all the world's starving people and to completely eliminate famine from the earth.

On a more individual level, studies have shown that vegetarians have greater stamina and long-term energy than meat eaters. Incidence of colon cancer and a number of other malignancies is lower in individuals who follow a vegetarian diet. And vegetarians have a sharply lower incidence of obesity, which is a major risk factor for hypertension, diabetes, and many other diseases. While animal foods contain toxins and metabolic waste products from the animal's own bodily processes, vegetarian foods are easier to digest because plants lack the complex physiologies of cattle or pigs. All in all, it's an inescapable conclusion that vegetarian foods are healthier and more efficient energy sources than animal foods.

One important recommendation of this chapter, therefore, is that you try to eliminate red meat from your diet altogether. Start by reducing the number of meals that include beef, pork, or veal, and try to substitute poultry, fish, or vegetarian foods. If you have already eliminated red meat from your diet or eat it only rarely, take the next step by reducing consumption of meat in any form, including poultry and seafood. Once you succeed in making several days each week completely meatless, I predict that you'll want to move toward a vegetarian diet, but this should be done at your own pace and according to your own day by day experience. By continuing to use your Energy Tracking Chart, you can see how reducing meat affects your energy levels. And remember that the Ayurvedic definition of a meatless diet does not exclude most dairy products. By adding milk, cottage cheese, yogurt, or lassi to your meals, you can easily create nutritious, delicious, but meat-free eating habits.

Other Energy Depressers

Aged or fermented foods have by definition undergone a prolonged devitalizing process, and these foods tend to depress the level of energy in your body. Try to reduce or avoid them, particularly sour cheeses such as Swiss and cheddar.

You should also try to become somewhat discriminating about sugar. While sugar has a deservedly bad reputation among health-conscious people, the real problem is with highly refined sugar rather than the natural raw variety. Processing removes certain important organic constituents that buffer the effect of sugar on your body; as a result, refined sugar is absorbed too rapidly or in a too concentrated form. This produces a physiological imbalance in the form of a "sugar high," which is soon followed by "post-sugar fatigue." Raw sugar, however, makes an excellent natural sweetener, especially when eaten in moderate amounts.

Like refined sugar, coffee and alcohol also provide a brief energy lift that soon changes to fatigue. Both these substances foster Vata imbalances with prolonged use. It's best to avoid alcohol altogether and to drink no more than one cup of coffee per day. If you feel in need of more coffee, try to substitute one of the many varieties of herbal tea.

Don't try to withdraw suddenly from each and every energy-depleting food. Reduce your consumption gradually, one food at a time, while keeping track of how you feel. Your increased energy will be so reinforcing that you'll naturally want to move toward a healthier diet. If you find yourself wanting one of the foods in the de-energizing category, try to eat it only at lunch time, when the digestive fire is sharpest and your body has its greatest ability to assimilate foods with mildly toxic properties. Red meat or aged cheese, for example, have a much more draining effect on your system if eaten at night than at midday.

VITAMINS

Many people with chronic fatigue look for relief in commercially produced vitamins and other food supplements. Yet all natural vitamins and minerals are amply available in well-balanced meals. Moreover, vitamins and minerals don't act alone; they work in concert with one another and with other organic components found in foods. If you isolate a few substances and take them in the form of a tablet or a syrup, you'll be unlikely to obtain the balanced proportion of these nutrients that nature intended. You may even cause some additional imbalance. It's much safer and more effective to get your nutrition from natural food sources, and it's also considerably less expensive.

THE SIX TASTES

In Ayurveda, the taste of food is an important indicator of its effect on the doshas and, therefore, on the whole mind/body system. Taste, after all, is the central experience of eating. Animals in the wild rely on taste (along with smell, which is closely related to taste) for their eating cues. They don't know anything about the U.S. Recommended Daily Allowance for calcium, iron, and protein, yet they survive with only taste to guide them toward a balanced diet. This is a subject that has been largely overlooked by modern nutrition, but Ayurveda emphasizes the role of taste in creating dietary balance.

Ayurveda recognizes six basic tastes in food. In order to have a completely balanced diet, you should experience each of these six tastes every day, and ideally at every meal. Each taste is an important stimulus to the doshas; absence of any one of them will eventually create an imbalance in the system.

The six tastes and some examples are:

Sweet: sugar, milk, butter, rice, bread pasta
Sour: yogurt, lemon, cheese
Salty: salt
Pungent: Spicy foods, ginger, hot peppers
Bitter: Spinach, other green leafy vegetables, turmeric
Astringent: beans, lentils, pomegranate

It should be obvious that the modern American diet provides plenty of sweet, sour, and salty tastes, but it is relatively weak in pungent, bitter, and astringent. By eating larger quantities of vegetables, many health-conscious people are now including more of the bitter and astringent tastes in their meals, but it's important to recognize that pungent or spicy foods are also essential to some extent. Such foods are especially valuable because they enliven metabolism, and ginger is even called the "universal medicine" in Ayurveda because of its effect in stimulating the digestive fire.

The Ayurvedic viewpoint on the six tastes is summarized by our next Primary Energy Principle:

PEP 13. Variety is the spice of life, and including all six tastes in the daily diet is crucial to creating balance and energy.

DIET, DIGESTION, AND THE DOSHAS

So far, the recommendations in this chapter apply to everyone regardless of body type. However, some individual foods can be beneficial or detrimental to Vata, Pitta, and Kapha, and familiarity with these foods can be very important to anyone experiencing chronic fatigue. The following PEP expresses this principle:

PEP 14. Because of the principle of biological individuality, different foods create balance or imbalance for different people, depending on their body type.

VATA-BALANCING FOODS

You'll recall that Vata is described as "airy and windy." It also has qualities of lightness, coldness, roughness, dryness, quickness, and changeability. To help balance Vata, we need foods of the opposite qualities—foods that are warm, heavy, and oily. Foods of sweet or sour taste also tend to have a balancing effect on Vata.

To create a Vata-balancing diet, follow the chart below.

VATA-BALANCING DIET

1. *Favor* foods that are warm, heavy, and oily.
   Minimize foods that are cold, dry, and light.
2. *Favor* foods that are sweet, sour, and salty.
   Minimize foods that are spicy, bitter, and astringent.
3. Eat larger quantities, but not more than you can digest easily.

SOME SPECIFIC RECOMMENDATIONS

- Dairy. All dairy products pacify Vata.
- Sweeteners. All sweeteners are good (in moderation) for pacifying Vata.
- Oils. All oils reduce Vata.
- Grains. Rice and wheat are very good. *Reduce* barley, corn, millet, buckwheat, rye, and oats.
- Fruits. Favor sweet, sour, or heavy fruits, such as oranges, bananas, avocados, grapes, cherries, peaches, melons, berries, plums, pineapples, mangoes, and papayas. *Reduce* dry or light fruits, such as apples, pears, pomegranates, and cranberries.

- **Vegetables.** Beets, cucumbers, carrots, asparagus, and sweet potatoes are good. They should be eaten cooked, not raw. The following vegetables are acceptable in moderate quantities if they're cooked, especially with ghee or oil and Vata-reducing spices: peas, broccoli, cauliflower, celery, zucchini, and green leafy vegetables. It's better to avoid sprouts and cabbage.
- **Spices.** Cardamom, cumin, ginger, cinnamon, salt, cloves, mustard seed, and small quantities of black pepper are good.
- **Nuts.** All nuts are good.
- **Beans.** ***Reduce*** all beans, except for tofu and split-mung bean soup.
- **Meat and fish** (for nonvegetarians). Chicken, turkey, and seafoods are all right. Beef should be avoided.

PITTA-BALANCING FOODS

Pitta is like fire. Its qualities are hot, sharp, slightly oily, and acidic. Foods that balance Pitta are cool but not cold, neither excessively oily nor dry, and neither extremely pungent nor sour. Very sour or fermented foods such as vinegar or certain citrus fruits are especially destabilizing to Pitta because of their acidic properties. Sour cheeses are also in this category, and even yogurt can be too sour for most Pitta types when eaten plain. For Pittas, yogurt is best taken in the form of lassi. Tomatoes and tomato sauces can also cause a marked increase in Pitta dosha.

To create a Pitta-balancing diet, follow the chart below.

PITTA-BALANCING DIET

1. *Favor* foods that are cool and liquid.
   Minimize foods that are hot in temperature.
2. *Favor* tastes that are sweet, bitter, or astringent.
   Minimize spicy, salty, or sour tastes.

SOME SPECIFIC RECOMMENDATIONS

- **Dairy.** Milk, butter, and ghee are good for pacifying Pitta. ***Reduce*** yogurt, cheese, sour cream, and cultured buttermilk (as their sour tastes aggravate Pitta).
- **Sweeteners.** All sweeteners are good except honey and molasses.
- **Oils.** Olive, sunflower, and coconut oils are best. ***Reduce*** sesame, almond, and corn oil, all of which increase Pitta.
- **Grains.** Wheat, white rice, barley, and oats are good. ***Reduce*** corn, rye, millet, and brown rice.
- **Fruits.** Favor sweet fruits, such as grapes, cherries, melons, berries, avocados, coconuts, pomegranates, mangoes, and sweet, fully ripened oranges, pineapples, and plums. ***Reduce*** sour fruits, such as grapefruits, olives, papayas, persimmons, and sour, unripe oranges, pineapples, and plums.
- **Vegetables.** Favor asparagus, cucumbers, potatoes, sweet potatoes, pumpkins, broccoli, cauliflower, celery, okra, lettuce, beans, green beans, zucchini, and green leafy vegetables such as lettuce. ***Reduce*** hot peppers, tomatoes, carrots, beets, onions, garlic, radishes, spinach, and mustard greens.
- **Beans.** ***Reduce*** all beans, except tofu and split-mung dhal.
- **Spices.** Cinnamon, coriander, cardamom, and fennel are good. But the following spices strongly increase Pitta and should be eaten only in small amounts: ginger, cumin, black pepper, fenugreek, clove, celery seed, salt, and mustard seed. Chili peppers and cayenne should be avoided.
- **Meat and fish** (for nonvegetarians). Chicken, pheasant, and turkey are preferable. Beef, seafood, and egg yolk increase Pitta and should be avoided.

KAPHA-BALANCING FOODS

Kapha is the earthy and watery dosha. It is heavy, stable, oily, slow, dull, and sweet. Foods that balance Kapha are light and dry, and the pungent, bitter, and astringent tastes are especially helpful for waking up and balancing Kapha dosha. Grains such as barley, millet, and corn are very beneficial, as are green leafy vegetables and almost all spices. But heavy, oily, and cold foods tend to aggravate Kapha.

If Kapha is your principal dosha, consult this chart in formulating your diet.

KAPHA-BALANCING DIET

1. *Favor* foods that are light, dry, and warm.
   Minimize foods that are heavy, oily, and cold.
2. *Favor* foods that are spicy, bitter, and astringent.
   Minimize foods that are sweet, salty, and sour.

SOME SPECIFIC RECOMMENDATIONS

- Dairy. In general, ***avoid*** dairy products, ***except*** low-fat milk.
- Fruits. Lighter fruits, such as apples and pears, are best. ***Reduce*** heavy or sour fruits, such as oranges, bananas, pineapples, figs, dates, avocados, coconuts, and melons, since these fruits increase Kapha.
- Sweeteners. Honey is excellent for reducing Kapha. ***Reduce*** sugar products, as these increase Kapha.
- Beans. All beans are fine ***except*** tofu, which increases Kapha.
- Nuts. ***Reduce*** all nuts.
- Grains. Most grains are fine, especially barley and millet. Avoid wheat and rice, as they increase Kapha.
- Vegetables. All are fine, ***except*** tomatoes, cucumbers, sweet potatoes, and zucchini, as they all increase Kapha.
- Spices. All spices are good except salt, which should be avoided, as it increases Kapha.
- Meat and fish (for nonvegetarians). White meat from chicken or turkey is fine, as is seafood. ***Reduce*** red meat.

TASTE AND THE DOSHAS

Just as certain foods have a balancing effect on specific body types, the various tastes can do so as well. The chart below describes the effects of each taste on the doshas.

HOW THE SIX TASTES INFLUENCE THE DOSHAS	
Decrease Vata	Sweet, sour, salty
Increase Vata	Pungent, bitter, astringent
Decrease Pitta	Sweet, bitter, astringent
Increase Pitta	Pungent, sour, salty
Decrease Kapha	Pungent, bitter, astringent
Increase Kapha	Sweet, sour, salty

Remember the guiding principle of trying to experience all six tastes every day, ideally at every meal. But there's no need to become anxious or rigid about it. Just use this information to help enhance your enjoyment of food.

Above all, you should have fun with your diet and with all these recommendations. Worrying about dietary rules will certainly not help your problem of fatigue, and could even exacerbate it. Your own tastes and preferences will provide excellent directions as to which foods your mind/body system needs, and as you come more into balance, you'll be increasingly able to trust your internal signals. As you grow in self-awareness, your enjoyment of food and of life in general will grow as well.

In closing, here's a brief summary of the recommendations made in this chapter.

1. Learn to recognize energizing and energy-depleting foods. Begin orienting your diet toward the former and away from the latter.
2. Become familiar with the six tastes and begin to incorporate them into your daily diet, ideally at every meal.

3. Read over the dosha-balancing diets provided in this chapter. Start bringing your diet into line with your body type. Try making a list of some foods you like that are beneficial to your dosha, and plan some meals that include these.
4. Continue to track your energy by completing an Energy Tracking Chart each day. Note any relationships between your eating experiences and your energy levels.
5. Most important, have fun with the knowledge you've gained and enjoy eating!

5

ELIMINATING FATIGUE BY REDUCING STRESS

So far we've been looking at biological causes of chronic fatigue, but there's evidence that the mind is an even more important influence in creating this problem. In chapter 1, I referred to a study published in the *Journal of the American Medical Association* that considered more than one thousand people suffering from chronic fatigue. Despite thorough physical examinations and blood tests, only a small minority of these people were found to have any physical abnormalities. But 80 percent of the chronic fatigue patients displayed recognizable symptoms of anxiety or depression.

YOUR BODY'S INTERNAL PHARMACY

The explanation for this once again can be found in the notion of a mind/body connection. This phenomenon is so obvious that it's amazing how modern medicine has managed to overlook it to a great extent. Now, however, the important role of neurochemicals and neuropeptides in physiology is finally beginning to be understood. These substances are brought into being whenever you have a thought or emotion. They then circulate throughout the body and adhere to every organ system. They are especially drawn to the digestive tract and to immune system cells, where they can have powerful energizing or energy-depleting effects.

Neurochemicals are often very powerful drugs. The category of neurochemicals called endorphins, for example, discovered about twenty years ago, are natural painkillers produced by the brain. The word *endorphin,* derived from the Greek, literally means "internally produced morphine," and the comparison between endorphins and morphine is by no means an exaggeration. Morphine is probably the most powerful painkilling drug used in medicine; it is a narcotic opiate closely related to heroin. But many endorphins are fifty to one hundred times more powerful than morphine. It is amazing to think that the body can produce such a potent painkiller, and yet it does so all the time in very small amounts, or even in larger amounts if acute pain is present.

Endorphins are one example of literally thousands of naturally occurring biochemicals that the brain produces in order to create health and healing. The great advantage of these natural, internally produced chemicals over drugs that you buy in a pharmacy is that our own neurochemicals are produced in just the right amount, at just the right time, in response to the body's perception of pain or some other biological need. And there are no side effects to these natural biochemicals, since they are part of the body's own natural healing system.

Just as it contains potent painkillers, the brain's natural pharmacy also contains compounds to reestablish balance in all the body's major systems, including its energy systems. Learning how to use the brain's pharmacy properly is literally the key to perfect health. By gaining mastery in this area, you'll be able to produce compounds that enhance your body's vital systems much more effectively than any pep pill or stimulant could. Of course, you'll also be able to shut down production of any neurochemicals that weaken the body's energy-producing and healing capabilities.

The brain's neurochemical production is controlled by the mind. Balance of mind will produce balance of the brain's chemistry, which will in turn promote optimum functioning of the body's energy systems. But how does one create balance of mind? The first step, and probably the most important, is to reduce and eliminate stress.

STRESS, DIGESTION, AND IMMUNE RESPONSE

Stress has become a familiar term. It calls up images of being caught on an expressway at rush hour, of hurrying to meet deadlines, of angry words and disappointments. Ayurveda defines stress as an "undue pressure of experience." This takes place when the mind/body system is subjected to events that it is not prepared to handle in a balanced and integrated way. The pressure of this experience has an overpowering influence on the physiology. We generally think of stress as being caused by unpleasant situations, but even a positive experience can impose "undue pressure" on the system. If you were informed that you'd just won twenty million dollars in the lottery, your heart would start to race, your blood pressure would shoot up, and you would break out in perspiration. These are signs of a stress reaction, and they're also manifestations of the mind/body connection—a purely physiological event has produced an immediate biological effect on the body. Psychologists call this the "fight-or-flight response," a term that may be familiar to you. In the fight-or-flight response, fear or anxiety gives rise to neurochemicals that circulate throughout the body and affect many different systems. In addition to increased heart rate, digestion shuts down and there may be a feeling of nausea as blood is shunted away from the stomach and intestines and into the muscles. Your hair may even stand on end.

The fight-or-flight response is a huge energy drain on the body. Even small versions of the response can take a toll, and these are elicited every day during the normal course of events. When life starts to feel like a constant battle, you can be sure that miniature versions of the fight-or-flight response are continually being elicited throughout the body.

In short, stress changes the body's ability to function efficiently. Long-term stress undermines the crucial energy-producing activities of digestion and elimination, and evidence for this can be found in common expressions like "My stomach was tied up in knots" or "I had a lump in my throat." If the body is constantly mobilizing energy into the muscles to deal with perceived crises, there is little strength left to process food. Chronic fatigue is the inevitable result.

In addition to its effects on digestion, stress weakens the immune system. Neurochemicals called immunomodulators are produced in the brain and have a direct impact on the functioning of immune system cells. More specifically, immunomodulators produced during the fight-or-flight response depress physiological defense systems so that individuals under chronic stress have weaker immunity than others. There has been considerable research seeking to link weakened immune response to Chronic Fatigue Syndrome, the severe form of fatigue discussed in chapter 1.

PEP number 15 summarizes the relationship between stress and fatigue:

> PEP 15. The stress response is a major factor in producing chronic fatigue. It does so by interfering with the body's energy-producing systems, especially digestion, and by weakening immune system defenses.

MEDITATION AND REDUCED STRESS

Stress can be eliminated by providing the system with experiences that are opposite to stress, such as deep relaxation, rejuvenating exercise, and rest. The techniques on the following pages are simple but very powerful means for accomplishing this.

The many benefits of meditation have been verified in study after study, and millions of people around the world can attest to the positive effects of this practice. Some forms of meditation include the use of mantras; these are primordial sounds that are subvocally repeated as a way of bringing heightened awareness to the mind. Primordial sound meditation is taught at the Center for Mind/Body Medicine in California and by other authorities, but it is far from the only useful meditation technique. The breathing meditation described below is easy to learn without outside instruction, and it provides extremely valuable stress-reducing benefits.

Breathing Meditation

1. Set aside a time when you can be free from interruptions and responsibilities.
2. Find a quiet room away from traffic noise or other distractions. Sit quietly on the floor or in a straight-back chair, and close your eyes.
3. Breathe normally, but as you exhale and inhale begin gradually directing your awareness toward your breathing. Without trying to control or influence it in any way, become aware of the coming and going of your breath.
4. If you notice your breath getting faster or slower, or even stopping altogether for a moment, just observe this without resistance or encouragement. Allow it to stabilize by itself.

5. If your thoughts distract you or you become unfocused in any way, don't resist. Just allow your attention to come back naturally to your breathing.
6. Continue this meditation for fifteen minutes. Then, still sitting with your eyes closed, allow another few minutes for gradual return to everyday consciousness.

As you gain experience with this technique, you'll find your thoughts becoming progressively quieter during meditation. Ultimately, your mind can settle down completely, enabling you to access the thoroughly tranquil state that precedes everyday thought. This sense of pure relaxation can be extremely important and valuable. Experiencing it on a regular basis will be tremendously beneficial in reducing stress and the fatigue that almost always accompanies it.

Use the Breathing Meditation twice a day, in the morning and the evening. Just as you've been doing with the changes in your diet, note the effects of meditation on your Energy Tracking Chart. Meditation is one of the safest and most effective methods for reducing stress and restoring energy, and the small amount of discipline it requires is sure to be greatly rewarded.

NEUROMUSCULAR AND NEURORESPIRATORY INTEGRATION

In addition to meditation, neuromuscular and neurorespiratory integration are mind/body techniques that can be extremely effective in reducing stress and fatigue.

Neuromuscular integration consists of a set of yoga stretching exercises that energize the relationships among the mind, the nervous system, and the other processes in the body. These are not exercises in the usual sense, which denotes strenuous physical activity. Neuromuscular integration is a more subtle practice, which is in fact quite effortless, and it works by enlivening certain vital points in the physiology that Ayurveda calls *marmas.*

There are 108 of these marma points, which are like control switches for directing energy and biological intelligence to various parts of the body. The purpose of the techniques presented here is to integrate the functioning of all the marma points in the body. When this takes place, a uniform and balanced flow of energy is established throughout the whole physiological system.

Neuromuscular Integration Exercises

The simple yoga postures that follow help restore mind/body coordination and balance at all levels. Each of the postures stretches a separate part of the body, thereby enlivening the marma present in the different areas. A key fact about neuromuscular integration is its *mind/body* character: the mental component of the activity is as important as the physical. It's very important to hold the posture for the recommended time period. While holding it, allow your awareness to rest easily on the area of the body that is being stretched. This will most likely happen by itself. You don't have to concentrate—just let your attention naturally gravitate to the area that's being exercised, and this will awaken the marma points in that area. The principle here is that of our first Primary Energizing Principle: Attention has organizing power. With the help of your attention, you can enlist the power of your body's natural healing mechanisms.

You should never allow yourself to feel any strain during these exercises. If you find that any of the postures are difficult or painful to achieve, you should avoid those exercises completely or perform them only in a limited way, stretching just to the point where you feel comfortable pressure but not strain. If you have any question about your ability to perform any or all of the postures without discomfort, it's best to consult a physician before proceeding. If you are in an older age group, or if you have any acute or chronic muscle, joint, or skeletal problems—chronic neck or back pain, for example—again it would be best to consult your doctor before undertaking the postures. Barring any of these conditions, you can do the neuromuscular integration exercises once or twice a day. The whole program takes about ten minutes to perform.

Begin by carefully reading these guidelines.

1. Be careful not to stretch farther than your body can easily accept. The illustrations depict the *ideal* execution of each posture, but you should stretch only to comfortable limits. With time, your flexibility will improve. If even minimal performance of a certain posture causes pain or discomfort, omit that posture. If you have back pain, or other chronic or acute muscular or skeletal problems, consult your physician before proceeding.
2. If you feel you can't bend a particular part of your body, don't force your body by swinging. Just bend to the extent you can, without force.
3. Hold each posture for the time indicated, and then release it easily. Breathe naturally during the exercises. Don't hold your breath.
4. Wear comfortable, loose clothing. Use a folded blanket, rug, or exercise mat to cushion a bare floor.
5. Don't perform the postures on a full stomach. Wait at least two or three hours after eating.
6. Allow your awareness to gravitate to the area that is being stretched. Your attention will naturally be drawn to that part of your body. By allowing it to rest there, you'll gain maximum benefit from the exercise.
7. These exercises take only about five minutes if you perform each posture once. If you have time, you can repeat each pose up to three times before starting the next one.
8. Be sure to perform the exercises in the order given, as each pose is designed to prepare your body for the next one.

1. TONING-UP EXERCISES

This two-minute body massage gently increases circulation, moving your blood in the direction of your heart.

1. Sit comfortably. Use the palms and fingers of both hands to press the top of your head, gradually moving toward your face, neck, and chest while press-ing and releasing. Then start again at the top of your head and gradually press and release down over the back of your neck and around to your chest.

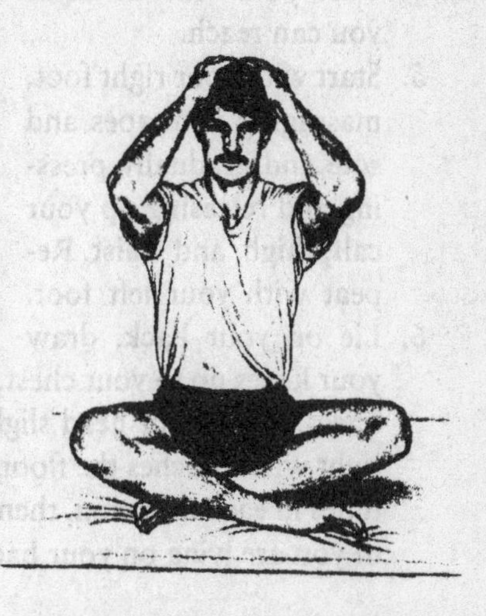

2. Grasp the fingertips of your right hand with the palm and fingers of your left hand, gradually pressing and releasing your arm up to your shoulder and chest. First do the upper side of your arm, then repeat on the underside. Then massage your left arm in the same way.

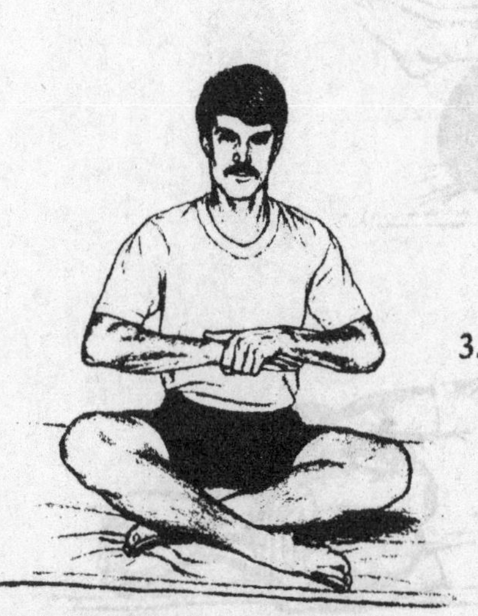

3. With the tips of your fingers meeting horizontally at the navel, begin to press and release your abdomen, gradually moving the pressure up toward your heart, reaching almost to your chest.

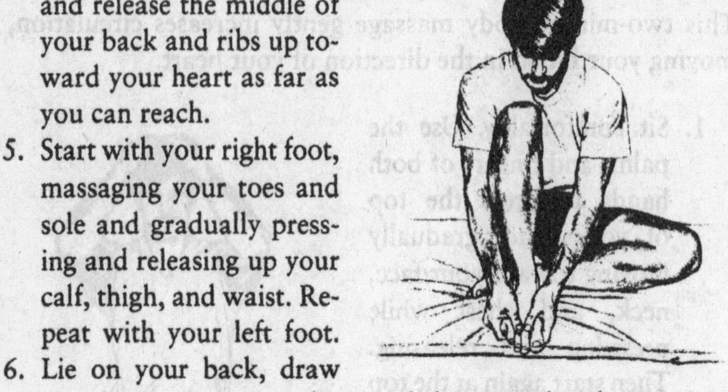

4. Use both hands to press and release the middle of your back and ribs up toward your heart as far as you can reach.
5. Start with your right foot, massaging your toes and sole and gradually pressing and releasing up your calf, thigh, and waist. Repeat with your left foot.
6. Lie on your back, draw your knees up to your chest, and clasp your hands over your knees. Raise your head slightly. Roll to the right until your right wrist touches the floor, then roll to the left. Repeat five times in each direction, then slowly stretch your legs out until you are lying on your back. Rest for a few seconds.

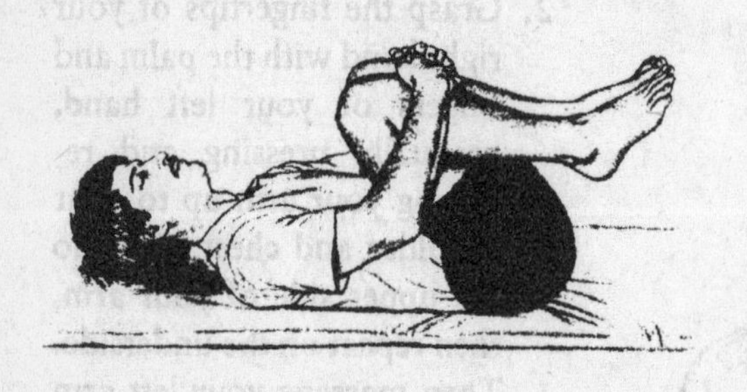

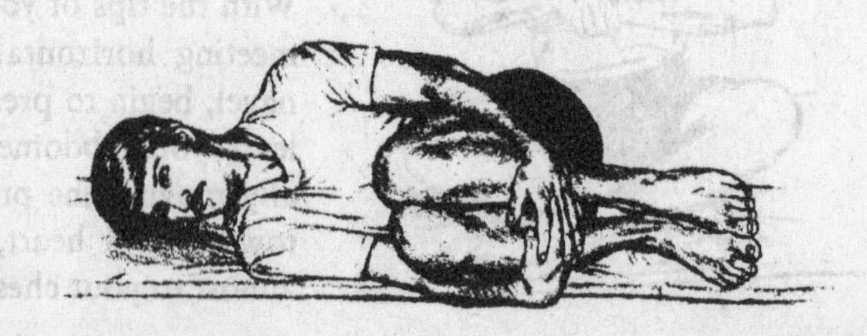

2. SEAT-STRENGTHENING POSE

This exercise prepares your body for the other postures, strengthening your pelvic area and back.

1. Kneel down, sitting on the flat of your feet, with heels apart and your big toes crossed. Place your hands in your lap, palms up. Hold your head, neck, and spine in a straight line.

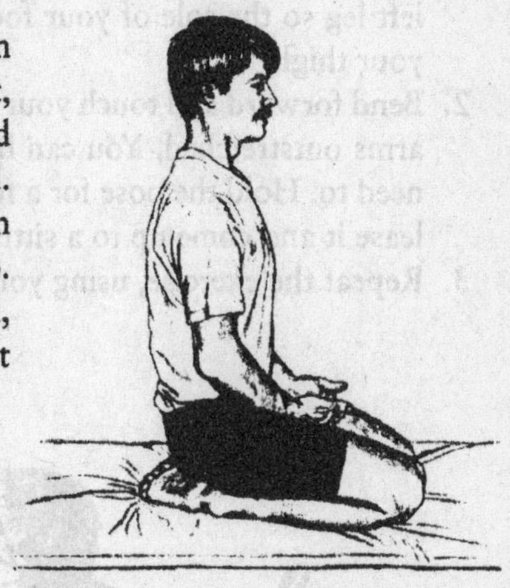

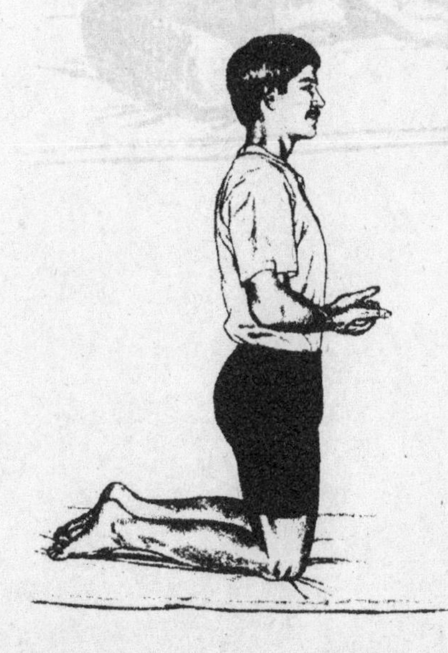

2. Next, lift your buttocks off your heels until you are in a kneeling position. Then slowly lower your body and sit down on your heels again. Repeat, moving slowly and smoothly.

3. Head-to-Knee Pose

This posture strengthens and relaxes your spine and abdominal organs, aiding digestion.

1. Sit and stretch your right leg in front of you. Bend your left leg so the sole of your foot is touching the inside of your thigh.
2. Bend forward and touch your right foot with your hands, arms outstretched. You can bend your right knee if you need to. Hold the pose for a few seconds, then slowly release it and come up to a sitting position.
3. Repeat the exercise, using your other leg.

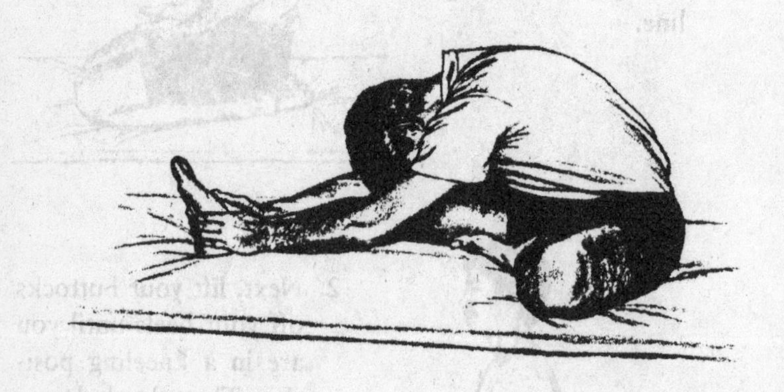

4. Shoulder Stand

This posture enlivens the endocrine system and the thyroid gland, relieves mental fatigue, makes your spine more flexible, and has a soothing effect on your body.

1. Lie on your back. Slowly raise your legs to a vertical position, over the waist. Support your back with your hands above your hips, keeping your elbows in toward your body.
2. Tilt your feet more toward your head. Hold the pose for half a minute.
3. Slowly return to the original position by bending your knees to balance your trunk until your buttocks touch the floor, then straighten your legs and lower them slowly. Relax gradually. Breathe normally and naturally throughout all the exercises.
4. Be careful not to strain your neck or throat—this is a shoulder stand, not a neck stand.

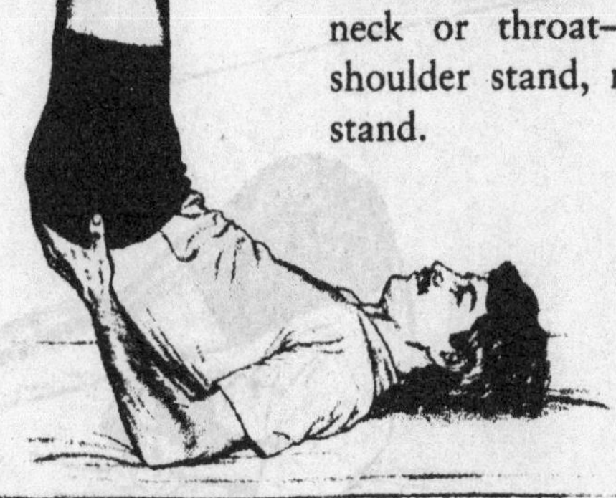

5. Plow Pose

This pose strengthens and relaxes your back, neck, and shoulders. It normalizes the functioning of the liver, spleen, and thyroid and removes fatigue.

1. From the shoulder stand, continue into this position as you bend from your pelvis and bring both legs down over your head.
2. Allow your legs to go back only as far as feels comfortable. Be careful not to put too much strain on your neck. Extend your arms straight out behind you. Your torso should rest on the tops of your shoulders, your hips maintaining a vertical line with your shoulder joints. Cross your arms over your head, holding this position for a few seconds.

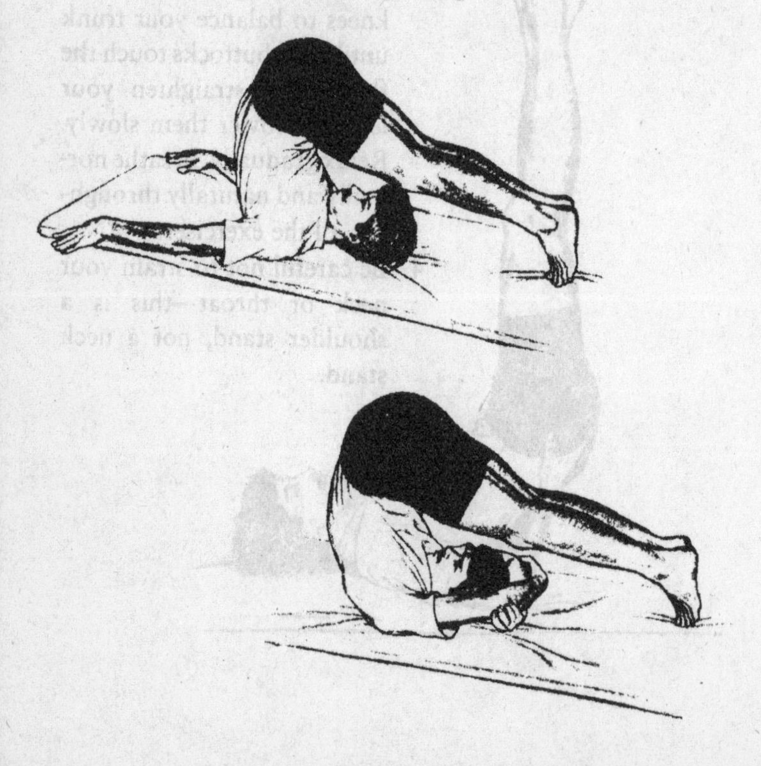

3. Slowly return to a prone position by bending your knees to balance your torso until your buttocks touch the floor. Then straighten your legs and lower them slowly. Relax.

6. COBRA POSE

This exercise strengthens and relaxes your back muscles and helps with irregularities in the ovaries and uterus.

1. Lie on your chest with your palms directly under your shoulders, fingers pointing forward. Place your forehead on the floor.
2. Slowly raise your head and chest, keeping your elbows close in to your body, and maintain the pose for a few seconds.
3. Bend your elbows, slowly lowering yourself until you are lying comfortably, resting your right or left cheek on the floor. Relax completely.

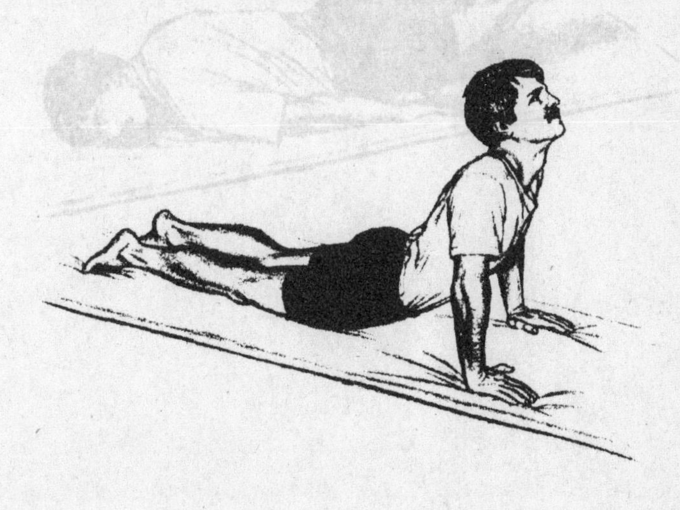

7. Locust Pose

This posture strengthens your lower back, aids in digestion, and balances the bladder, prostate, uterus, and ovaries.

1. Continue to lie on your chest, with your arms along the sides of your body, palms up. Let your chin rest gently on the floor.
2. Raise your legs in a straight position, extending them upward and back. Hold the pose for a few seconds while breathing easily. Then release your legs slowly.
3. If you find it difficult to raise both legs together in the beginning, do not strain. Try raising one leg at a time.

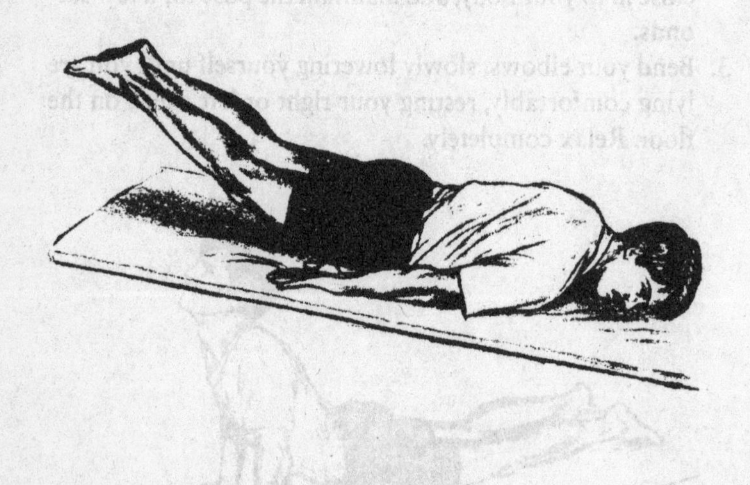

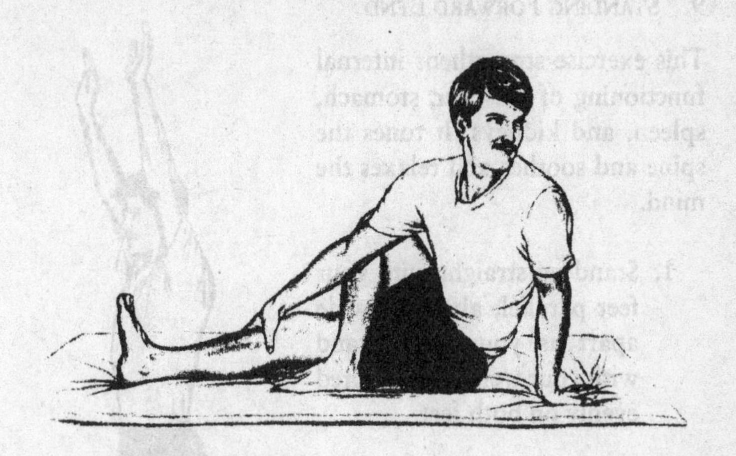

8. SEATED TWIST POSE

This pose increases circulation in the liver, spleen, adrenal glands, and kidneys. It also releases tightness in the shoulders, upper back, and neck.

1. Sit with your legs stretched out in front of you.
2. Raise your left leg so that your foot is on the floor near your right knee.
3. Put your left hand on the floor behind you.
4. Gently turn your torso to the left, press your right forearm against the outside of your left knee, and grasp your right leg below the knee.
5. Turn your head and torso to your left.
6. Maintain the pose for a few seconds and come back slowly to the original seated position. Repeat the pose with your other leg.

9. Standing Forward Bend

This exercise strengthens internal functioning of the liver, stomach, spleen, and kidneys. It tones the spine and soothes and relaxes the mind.

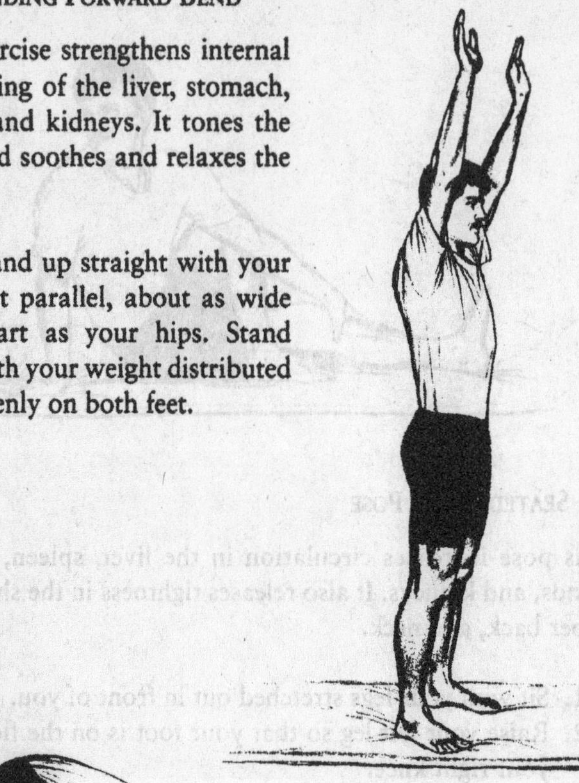

1. Stand up straight with your feet parallel, about as wide apart as your hips. Stand with your weight distributed evenly on both feet.

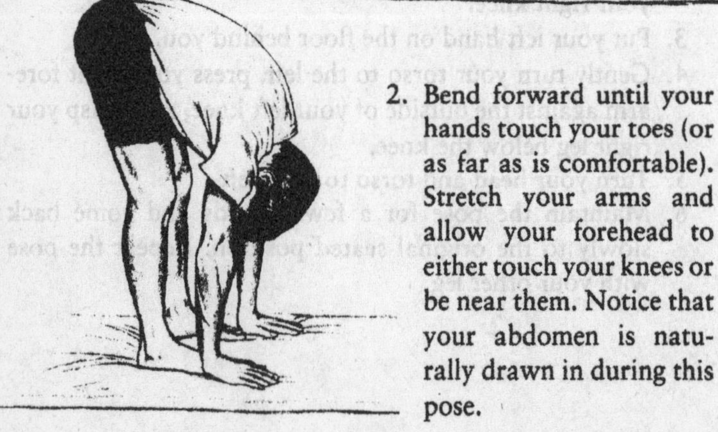

2. Bend forward until your hands touch your toes (or as far as is comfortable). Stretch your arms and allow your forehead to either touch your knees or be near them. Notice that your abdomen is naturally drawn in during this pose.

10. AWARENESS POSE

This soothing pose eliminates fatigue and rejuvenates the body and mind.

1. Lie on your back, allowing your arms to rest easily by your sides with your palms up.
2. Allow your body to relax. Close your eyes and let your awareness be easily drawn to any part of your body or to your body as a whole.
3. Rest for at least one minute, breathing easily and naturally.

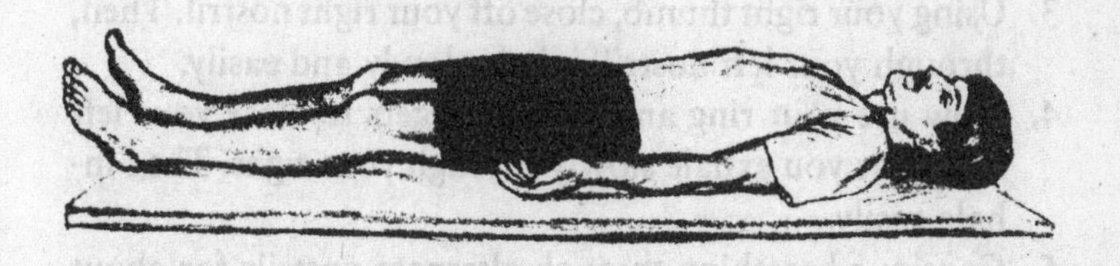

Neurorespiratory Integration

Breathing is every bit as important as digestion in the production of physiological energy, because energy is produced when oxygen is combined with food. Therefore the quality of our respiration is very influential in how energetic we feel. When breathing is balanced and relaxed, it promotes vitality throughout the system. But if respiration is shallow or unbalanced, the body doesn't get the full complement of vital energy it needs.

Ayurveda recognizes the important relationship between breathing and vitality. The Ayurvedic word Prana means "vital breath," and a whole area of Ayurvedic science, called Pranayam is devoted to creating balanced respiration. The more specific term Pranayama refers to neurorespiratory integration exercises that help to develop good breathing habits.

The Pranayama technique introduced here is easy to perform, takes only about five minutes, and can be an excellent revitalizer. It involves alternating your breathing between each nostril. During the practice of this technique, you should breathe a little more deeply and a little more slowly than you do during normal restful breathing. Some people may find it a bit confusing at first, so please read the instructions carefully:

1. Sit easily and comfortably with your spine as straight as possible.
2. Close your eyes and rest your *left* hand on your knee. For this part of the exercise you will be using your thumb and the middle and ring fingers of your *right* hand.
3. Using your right thumb, close off your right nostril. Then, through your left nostril, inhale slowly and easily.
4. Now use your ring and middle fingers to close your left nostril as you exhale slowly through your right. Then inhale easily.
5. Continue breathing through alternate nostrils for about five minutes. Your breathing may be slightly slower and deeper than usual, but it should be natural and unforced.
6. When you're done, sit quietly for a few minutes as you breathe easily and normally.

This neuromuscular integration technique balances air flow between the left and right hemispheres of the brain, thus integrating mind and body. Modern physiology has revealed that the two hemispheres have very different functions: the left relates principally to linear reasoning and to linguistic and mathematical skills, while the right controls imaginative and intuitive functions such as spatial orientation and creative thinking. Stimulation of the inner lining of the nostrils by alternating the air flow sends sequential impulses to the two brain hemispheres. This helps to integrate their respective functions and to produce neurophysiological balance. The ultimate effect is to wake up the whole system, creating greater mental and physical energy.

The techniques presented so far in this chapter should be undertaken in a specific sequence. The neuromuscular integration exercises should be performed first, followed by the neurorespiratory technique. Breathing meditation should come last. This creates a progression from a grosser level (the body) to a more subtle level (breathing) to the most subtle level of all, which is the mind. If you don't have time for all three techniques in succession, you may of course do any one of them alone. If you have to choose, meditation would be the most valuable.

AYURVEDIC OIL MASSAGE

Daily oil massage is a traditional part of the Ayurvedic routine. The massage takes roughly five to ten minutes, and it should be performed each morning before your shower or bath as a way of purifying and balancing the entire physiology. It can even be done in as little as two or three minutes.

The Ayurvedic oil massage balances Vata dosha throughout the system. Because Vata is light, cold, and dry, a massage using warm oil can have a soothing and pacifying effect. This is significant because Vata is easily unbalanced by stress, and chronic fatigue soon results. In addition, the massage stimulates circulation and helps remove impurities from the whole body.

Here are the instructions for performing the Ayurvedic oil massage, together with information on how to heat sesame oil, which Ayurveda considers to have a uniquely balancing and vitalizing influence. Briefly heating the oil energizes it, helps to thin it out, and facilitates its absorption into the body. Be sure to follow the instructions carefully.

How to Do Ayurvedic Oil Massage

It's ideal to do Ayurvedic oil massage in the morning, before your shower or bath.

1. Start with cold-pressed sesame oil, available from your health food store. Ideally, the oil should be cured (purified) before using. (Instructions for curing are given below.) The oil should be warmed each day before you use it. One easy way to do this is to keep the oil in a small plastic bottle with a flip-top lid. Warm the oil by placing the bottle in a sink filled with hot water for a few minutes.
2. Use the open part of your hand, rather than your fingertips, to massage your entire body. In general, use circular motions over rounded areas (joints, head) and straight strokes over straight areas (neck, long bones). Apply moderate pressure over most of your body and light pressure over your abdomen and heart.
3. Start with your head. Pour a small amount of oil on your hands and vigorously massage it into your scalp. With the flat part of your hands, use circular strokes to cover your whole head. Spend more time massaging your head than other parts of your body.
4. Next, massage your face and outer ears, remembering to apply a small amount of oil as you move from one part of your body to the next. Massage this area more gently.
5. Massage the front and back of your neck and the upper part of your spine. At this point you may want to cover the rest of your body with a thin layer of oil to give it maximum time to soak in.
6. Vigorously massage your arms, using a circular motion on your shoulders and elbows and long, back-and-forth strokes on your upper arms and forearms.
7. Now massage your chest and stomach. Use a very gentle, circular motion over your heart and abdomen. You can

start in the lower right part of your abdomen and move clockwise toward the lower left part, to gently massage your intestines.

8. Massage your back and spine. You may have trouble reaching your entire back. Just do the best you can.
9. Massage your legs vigorously, using circular motions over your hips, knees, and ankles. Use long, straight strokes over your thighs and calves.
10. Finally, massage the bottoms of your feet. As with your head, this important area of your body deserves more time. Use the palm of your hand to massage your soles vigorously.
11. Follow your oil massage with a warm bath or shower, using a mild soap.

How to Prepare Sesame Oil for Ayurvedic Oil Massage

Ayurveda recommends using unprocessed, cold-pressed sesame oil, which is available at health food stores. Before using the sesame oil, cure the oil by following these simple steps. Curing increases the oil's ability to penetrate the skin.

1. Heat the oil to about the boiling temperature of water (212° F). To know when the oil is hot enough, simply add a single drop of water to the oil before you heat it. When the water crackles or boils on top of the oil, you can remove it from the heat. Or just observe the oil as it heats. When it begins to move and circulate in the pan, remove it from the burner.
2. If you like, you can cure up to one quart of oil at a time. This should be enough for at least two weeks.
3. **Caution:** Because all oils are flammable, be sure to observe proper safety precautions. Use low rather than high heat, never leave the room while the oil is heating, and re-

move it promptly once the proper temperature is reached. Be sure to store it in a safe place when cooling, out of reach of children.

It's best to perform the massage every day, but many people initially find this difficult. I recommend that you start with one or two mornings a week. As with other mind/body techniques, it's likely that you'll feel so much better on the days when you've done the massage that you'll begin doing it more and more often, until you spontaneously find yourself doing it every day.

Please write down the following Primary Energy Principle, which summarizes the information in this chapter:

> PEP 16. To reduce fatigue, stress should be replaced by relaxation and rest. This can be accomplished through breathing meditation, neuromuscular and neurorespiratory integration techniques, and the Ayurvedic oil massage.

Having given considerable attention to the very important relationship between energy and the mind, we'll now consider how physical activity can enliven or deplete energy resources. This will be the subject of chapter 6.

6

Using Natural Rhythms to Create Energy

Every human being is part of the natural continuum. Nature's energy flows through us, and if we are skillful partners with the universe that surrounds us, we can make good use of that infinite reservoir of vitality and strength.

The intimate relationship between nature and each individual can be made dramatically clear through the study of biological rhythms. Ayurveda recognized thousands of years ago that nature operates in cycles, and that these cycles have a profound effect upon individual physiologies. More recently, modern physiology has identified many of the rhythms that influence our mind/body systems. We actually have many different "biological clocks" within us, each regulating different bodily functions according to precise time cycles. The most important of our internal tempos is called "circadian rhythm" by modern science. This is a twenty-four-hour cycle that controls many important processes, including body temperature, the production of hormones and other biochemicals, and nervous system functions such as waking and sleeping. The circadian rhythm has a number of important implications for chronic fatigue. The hormone cortisol, for example, which is produced by the adrenal glands, is a powerful anti-stress agent. Its presence in the body rises and falls according to a predictable pattern within each twenty-four-hour period. Cortisol levels in the blood reach their peak at the start of the day, around 7:00 A.M. They're at a low point in the late afternoon or early evening—a time when nature intends for our activities to ease off—and they remain low throughout the night. Body temperature follows a somewhat different twenty-four-hour cycle. It increases throughout the day, reaches a high point in the late afternoon or early evening, and then begins to decrease toward its low point a few hours after midnight.

There are also monthly and seasonal biological rhythms, such as the female menstrual cycle. And there are even cycles that occur according to the ebb and flow of the ocean tides. In short, the laws that govern our physical and emotional ups and downs are fundamentally inseparable from the larger rhythms of the world and even of the cosmos. They are all expressions of the same unified field of intelligence.

As a result of biological rhythms, "Timing is everything." There are times when it's appropriate to engage in certain activities, and other times when those same activities are likely to be unproductive. With regard to chronic fatigue, an activity performed at a particular hour may help to enhance energy and physiological balance, while at a different time it could actually have a weakening effect.

> PEP 17. From a biological perspective, timing is everything. An activity performed at a certain time may promote balance and energy, while at a different moment that same activity can create imbalance and fatigue.

As the importance of biological rhythms has come to be recognized, it has created a whole new specialty in medical research known as chronobiology. Experiments in this field have confirmed the importance of proper timing. Studies in which mice have been exposed to high doses of radiation, for example, have demonstrated radically different survival rates depending on the time in which radiation was administered. These studies have important ramifications for many medical procedures, including X-rays and the chemical therapies used to treat cancer.

Biological rhythms are like waves of nature that are constantly passing over us. As if riding a surfboard, you should time your activities to "catch" these waves, and then allow yourself to be carried along on their crests. This creates energy and joy. Fighting the waves by challenging the natural cycles is like trying to stand up on a surfboard at the wrong time. A "wipeout" is inevitable—and, in terms of your energy, wiped out is exactly how you'll feel.

DAILY ENERGY CYCLES

Ayurveda long ago evolved a view of an optimum daily routine that recognizes the various phases of the twenty-four-hour cycle—and as you might expect, these phases are described in terms of Vata, Pitta, and Kapha. The alternating influence of the three doshas during each day has a distinct effect on how you feel and on how efficiently you're able to perform any activity.

As you can see, the Kapha influence is dominant from 6:00 A.M. until mid-morning. Then Pitta is dominant until mid-afternoon, and you'll recall that the digestive fire is at its peak during this time. This cycle of the doshas ends with a primarily Vata influence from 2:00 P.M. until sunset, whereupon a second cycle begins, which is similar to the first.

MASTER CYCLES OF VATA, PITTA, AND KAPHA

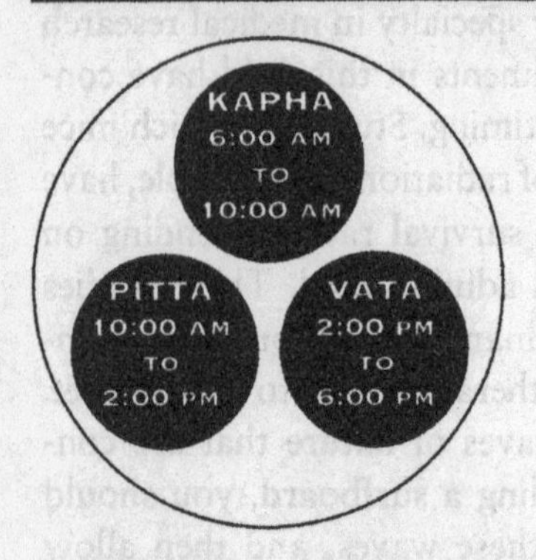

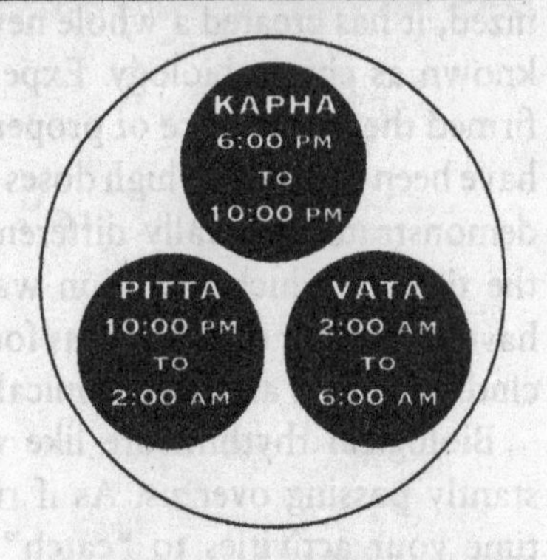

FIRST CYCLE

Kapha predominates from
6:00 A.M. to 10:00 A.M.
Pitta predominates from
10:00 A.M. to 2:00 P.M.
Vata predominates from
2:00 P.M. to 6:00 P.M.

SECOND CYCLE

Kapha predominates from
6:00 P.M. to 10:00 P.M.
Pitta predominates from
10:00 P.M. to 2:00 A.M.
Pitta predominates from
2:00 A.M. to 6:00 A.M.

So the twenty-four-hour day is divided into halves—daytime and nighttime—each of which contains three phases of the doshas. Within each cycle, Kapha appears first, then Pitta, and Vata last.

The influence of these dosha periods is obvious in the natural environment. In the evening, after work is completed and as the sun is setting, there's a sense of gathering silence, as if all of nature is settling down. There's a noticeable impulse to just sit back and relax as nightfall begins. Of course, if you live in a large metropolitan area you may wonder where this silence might be as you look out on ceaseless urban activity. Such activity, however, does not spring from any influence inherent in nature itself; rather, it is an artifact of the contemporary lifestyle, which often brings us into direct conflict with nature. But if you allow yourself to follow the naturally ordained influence of Kapha that dominates this period of the day, you'll feel relaxed, heavy, and inclined toward sleep.

Indeed, the ideal bedtime occurs at the junction point of the Kapha and Pitta periods of the evening, at 10:00 P.M. If you postpone going to sleep much beyond this point—beyond 11:00 P.M. for example—you'll miss the rejuvenating rest that best begins at the end of the Kapha cycle. Sleep that begins later will be lighter and imbued with restless Pitta qualities. Over time, a sleep cycle that is out of harmony with basic natural rhythms will necessarily lead to chronic fatigue.

Don't underestimate the importance of the sleep cycle. It can be an extremely significant source of energy once it's brought into balance.

THE RHYTHMS OF SLEEPING AND WAKING

Going to bed at the evening junction point of Kapha and Pitta is one of the keys to a balanced daily routine. Another equally important key is to wake up at the end of the Vata period in the morning, at the junction of Vata and Kapha. This occurs at sunrise, or around 6:00 A.M. When you awaken at this time, your mind and body are under the influence of Vata qualities such as lightness, quickness, alertness, enthusiasm, and exhilaration. This is simply the right time to start the day. But if you miss this natural waking point and sleep into the next phase of the morning, you'll wake up imbued with Kapha qualities of heaviness, dullness, and slowness. If this becomes your habitual sleep pattern, your physiological system will become chronically sluggish. There will be a smothering effect on all the body's energy-producing systems.

So you should go to bed early, and you should wake up early too. If this seems like an impossible price to pay for overcoming chronic fatigue, let me offer some practical suggestions.

First, recognize the obvious fact that your bedtime and your waking time are mutually dependent. In order to wake up early, it's very helpful to have gone to bed before ten o'clock the night before, and an early bedtime depends upon having evening activities that are conducive to relaxation. As we've seen, this is a time when nature intends us to ease off from strenuous activity in favor of a more restful mode. Dinner should be a relatively light meal. It should be eaten early, ideally at about 6:00 P.M., or by 7:00 at the latest; digestion will then be mostly completed by 10:00 P.M. Since digestion requires an increase in metabolism, it tends to disrupt sleep.

After dinner, try to enjoy light activities such as reading, spending time with your family, or talking with friends. Television is not particularly recommended because the electronic visual stimulus of the TV screen is intrinsically exciting to the nervous system, even if the content of a program is low-key. If watching TV in the evening is a daily ritual and it seems impossible to give this up, at least try to avoid it after 8:30 or 9:00 P.M. This will give the system an hour to settle down before bedtime. Likewise, if you find that you must do focused work at night, try to ease off such work by 9:00 P.M.

Just before bed you may find it helpful to drink something that will calm Vata dosha. A little warm milk with some Vata-pacifying herbs, such as a couple of pinches of cardamom and a small bit of saffron, makes a very nice bedtime drink. Nutmeg is another widely available spice that can be used instead of cardamom. If you have a problem with milk digestion, remember to add a pinch or two of fresh grated ginger prior to boiling the milk.

Your bedroom should be a sleeping room; watching TV or working in the bedroom should be avoided by all means. The decor of the bedroom should be restful, relaxing, and orderly, for a soothing influence on the system.

If you've gotten into bed by 10:00 P.M. but find that you're unable to sleep, resist the temptation to get up and read until you feel sleepier. Such an activity would have an aggravating influence on Vata dosha and would throw the system further out of synchrony with nature. Instead, simply continue to rest with your eyes closed, and adopt what I call a "not minding" attitude. This means recognizing that falling asleep is not really under your control, but is completely in nature's hands. Trying to fall asleep only interferes with the process. Biological rhythms like falling asleep operate according to what modern science calls the Law of Least Action: More activity on your part brings a less desirable result: So don't think about the process, and turn your clock to the wall. Your body will still get valuable needed rest. Although the effects of long-standing habits and disturbed biological rhythm may cause difficulty in falling asleep, it's much better to be in bed with the lights out during this early part of the night than to be up and about. You may initially feel uncomfortable, but by continuing to let your body rest at this period in the evening you'll soon begin to feel much better when you wake up. And your chronic fatigue will steadily improve as you grow accustomed to falling asleep during the Kapha period of the evening.

You'll most likely need an alarm clock in order to awaken at an early hour, at least while your system is adjusting to the new schedule. Choose an alarm that won't jolt you awake; I recommend a clock-radio tuned to a classical music station. Set the alarm for 6:00 A.M. or earlier, or 7:00 at the very latest. You should always get out of bed at this time, no matter how little sleep you think you've gotten or how tired you feel. Just get on with your daily activities—studies show that sleep deprivation from insomnia rarely interferes with most work-related tasks. Then, if you feel sufficiently tired in the evening, you'll naturally want to go to bed early.

In order to reset your biological clock in tune with natural rhythms, you must faithfully follow the plan of early-to-bed-early-to-rise. This includes weekends, holidays, and vacations, because even occasional wide variations in your sleep schedule can unbalance biological rhythms.

RECOMMENDATIONS FOR IMPROVING SLEEP

Sleeping in accord with natural cycles does more than provide extra rest; it also promotes what I call "blissful sleep." Blissful sleep comes from living in harmony with nature, and it is deeply refreshing and rejuvenating for the whole human system. It strengthens all the body's energy producing mechanisms, and it is one of your most valuable tools for ending chronic fatigue.

1. Try going to bed by 10:00 P.M. and rising by 6:00 A.M. on a regular basis.
2. To prepare your body for deep, restful sleep, follow these recommendations:
   - Eat a light, early dinner—by 6:00 P.M. or 7:00 P.M. at the latest—so you can completely digest your food before you go to bed.
   - Avoid focused work at night. Try to ease off by 9:00 P.M.
   - Plan relaxed evening activities, ideally with family or friends. Avoid watching TV, which overstimulates the nervous system.
   - Drink warm milk before bed. If you wish, add soothing spices such as cardamom, nutmeg, or saffron, which pacify Vata dosha.
   - Avoid working, reading, or watching TV in the bedroom, which should be exclusively for sleeping.
3. If you can't fall asleep immediately, adopt a calm "not minding" attitude. Don't get out of bed. Even if you aren't sleeping, your body is getting valuable rest.
4. If your bedtime and waking times have become widely out of tune with natural rhythms, try setting your alarm progressively earlier. Every three or four days, move your waking time ahead by ten or fifteen minutes. Gradually you'll start to feel sleepy earlier in the evening.

ELIMINATION

We've seen the importance of timing in fundamental processes such as digestion and sleep. We should also consider another basic biological function, that of elimination. There's no question that millions of people suffer from irregularities in their bowel movements, and once again the reason for this is found in the mind/body connection. More specifically, irregularity results from the effects of stress on gastrointestinal function.

The best time to have a bowel movement is shortly after awakening. This allows the body to rid itself of impurities from the previous day, so that the new day's activities are begun by a purified physiology.

Even if you have had problems in this area for a long time, you can retrain your system toward regularity. The most important principle is simply to take the time to allow bowel function to happen in an unforced way. After awakening, drink one or two glasses of warm water. Then go to the bathroom and just spend five to ten relaxed minutes, allowing bowel function to take place by itself. It's best, by the way, to avoid reading during this time. Reading will focus your attention upward or outward at a time when you want it to go inward and downward.

If nothing seems to be happening after ten minutes, get up and go about your business. But if you follow this procedure every day—intending to have a bowel movement but not minding whether you do or not—your body will begin to recapture nature's rhythm. Your system's purification mechanisms will become more integrated with natural cycles, and you'll experience the extra energy and clarity that this brings.

If you continue to have problems with constipation or other abnormalities of bowel function, I recommend another book in the Perfect Health Library, entitled *Perfect Digestion: The Key to Balanced Living*.

EXERCISES FOR THE THREE BODY TYPES

VATA

Slow-paced, light exercise that keeps the body in motion for 15 to 20 continuous minutes is best. Suggested exercises include walking, swimming, yoga exercises, and light bicycling.

PITTA

Brisker-paced but moderate exercise that keeps your body in motion for 15 to 20 continuous minutes is best. Suggested exercises include brisk walking, moderate cross-country skiing, swimming, cycling, weight lifting, tennis, and racquetball.

KAPHA

Vigorous exercise that lasts 15 to 30 minutes is best. You might try jogging, vigorous bicycling, swimming, cross-country skiing, aerobic workouts, walking, and heavy weight lifting.

AYURVEDIC GUIDELINES FOR HELTHY EXERCISE

- In general, use only 50 percent of your capacity. For example, if you are capable of running a maximum of six miles, run only three. Or if you can swim twelve laps at most, stop after six. Then you will feel energetic and comfortable, never strained or tired. And with regular exercise, your capacity will grow.
- Exercise every day, seven days a week.
- Do not strain when you exercise. If you start to breathe heavily through the mouth or start perspiring, cut back for now and then gradually increase the amount of exercise. Remember: No strain produces maximum gain.
- In general, exercise should be performed during the Kapha cycle in the morning (6:00 A.M. to 10:00 A.M.). If you practice meditation, it is best to exercise just afterward. However, the neuromuscular integration exercises and the Sun Salute, described below, are ideal techniques for settling the mind, and they should be performed prior to meditation.

EXERCISE AND THE DOSHAS

This is the final major element of the Ayurveda daily routine. One of the classic Ayurveda texts declares: "By physical exercise one gets lightness, capacity to work, firmness, tolerance of difficulties, diminution of physical impurities and strengthening of digestion and metabolism." In other words, exercise creates energy. But this quote is followed by another, equally important point: "Exercise should be performed in moderation."

The current emphasis on vigorous, strenuous, and generally *difficult* exercise is one reason why millions of people have so much trouble introducing regular physical activity into their lives. While vigorous exercise may be appropriate for certain body types, it has unpleasant effects on others, and this turns them away from exercise in general. This is unfortunate, since some form of moderate physical activity, in tune with your body type, is one of the most valuable things you can do to promote energy.

For Vata types, light exercise is definitely best. Vata, which is light and airy by nature, will not tolerate extremely strenuous activity. Such exercise will only lead to a Vata imbalance and to more fatigue. Walking and comparable activities, such as light swimming or bicycle riding, are the best choices for Vata types. Try to walk for fifteen or twenty minutes every day, easily but continuously. As tolerance increases, pace can also be increased until you're moving quite briskly. In addition to walking and equivalent exercises, the yoga postures of the neuromuscular integration program, which were introduced in chapter 5, can be of great benefit to Vata types.

Pitta types have moderate stamina, so they should engage in moderate forms of exercise. Activities involving continuous motion for at least fifteen to twenty minutes are best. For Pittas, however, the pace can be a bit more intense than for Vatas. Brisk walking, cycling, light to moderate weight lifting, cross-country skiing, and swimming are all good. Pittas also tend to enjoy competitive sports because of their dynamic and competitive natures. These activities are fine as long as the competition doesn't intensify to a point that inflames Pitta's aggressive tendencies. Games such as tennis or basketball involve more starting and stopping than continuous action and have less physiological value than continuous-motion types of exercise.

Kapha types, who incline toward heaviness, are the only individuals who benefit from really vigorous exercise. In its absence, Kaphas can easily become physically sedentary and mentally lazy. If you're a Kapha type, your tendency toward inertia can make it hard for you to get going, but the right kind of exercise will make you feel so much better that you'll soon gain momentum and enjoyment. Kapha-appropriate exercises include jogging, vigorous bicycling, swimming, or cross-country skiing, heavier weight lifting, and aerobic dance. Indoor exercise equipment can be helpful during the winter months to keep up a Kapha's more demanding exercise program.

Regardless of your body type, the best time for exercise is during the Kapha period of morning. This helps to lighten up Kapha and get the day off to a dynamic start. If you can't exercise in the morning, you can still do so anytime during the daytime hours; exercise after sundown isn't recommended, however, since it tends to agitate the system at a time when the body naturally wants to be settling down before bed.

Sun Salute

There is one kind of exercise in Ayurveda that is recommended for all body types and has a particularly energizing effect on the system. This exercise is called Surya Namaskara in Sanskrit or, in English, Sun Salute. It is traditionally performed in the early morning while facing the rising sun.

The Sun Salute comprises twelve postures that are alternated at roughly five-second intervals. A recommended breathing pattern accompanies the poses.

If you're not used to stretching, you may find it best to perform the neuromuscular integration exercises described in chapter 5 for a few weeks before undertaking the more vigorous Sun Salute. And if you're in an older age group or have any muscle or orthopedic problems, it's best to consult your doctor before doing this exercise.

Follow these general guidelines for the sun salute:

1. When you do the Sun Salute, allow a half-hour before a meal and three hours after a meal. If you practice other meditation programs or yoga postures, the Sun Salute can be performed before them.
2. One cycle of the Sun Salute, consisting of twelve postures, is described below. Start with as many cycles as is comfortable, and gradually increase to a maximum of twelve. Do not strain. If you start to breathe heavily or begin perspiring, lie down and rest for a minute or two.
3. Hold each position for about five seconds. The Eight Limbs Position (position 6) is the only exception, as it is held only one second.
4. The Sun Salute uses a specific pattern of breathing—inhale or exhale—for each posture. You will be instructed to inhale during *extension* postures—because inhaling facilitates the extending and lengthening movements of the spine. You will be asked to exhale on the *flexion* postures, because this helps the body to fold, bend, and flex.
5. You'll see that there are two Equestrian positions per cycle. Use the same knee forward during the same cycle. Switch to the opposite knee for the next cycle, and continue alternating with each new cycle. Always do an even number of cycles so that both sides of your body are exercised in a balanced way.
6. Do not rush through exercises; maximum value comes from doing them slowly. Each cycle takes one to two minutes.

7. After completing the final cycle, lie down on your back, arms at your sides, with palms facing upward, for two minutes. Just allow your attention to be easily on your body.
8. Be careful not to strain by stretching too far. The drawings show the ideal performance of each pose, but you should stretch only as far as your body is comfortable. Over time, more flexibility will develop. You should definitively not feel pain or discomfort while doing these exercises. If even minimal performance of a particular posture causes discomfort, omit that posture. If you have back problems, consult your physician before starting these exercises.

How to Do the Sun Salute

1. Salutation Position

Start the Sun Salute with your feet parallel and your weight distributed evenly over your feet. Place your hands together, palms touching, at chest level. Breathe easily for about five seconds.

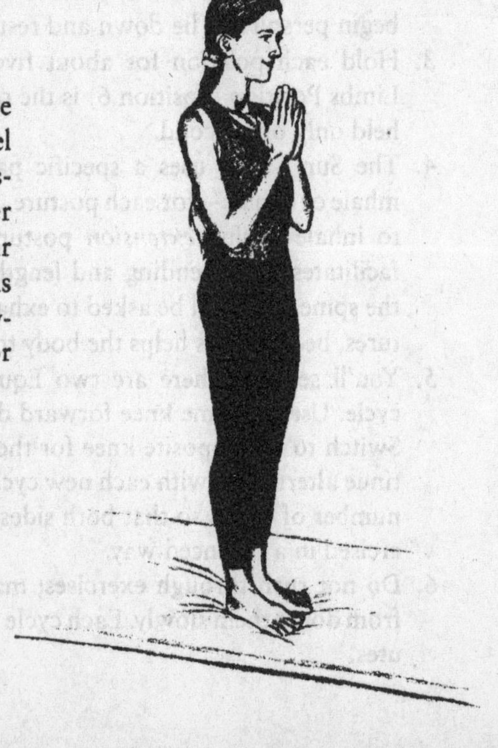

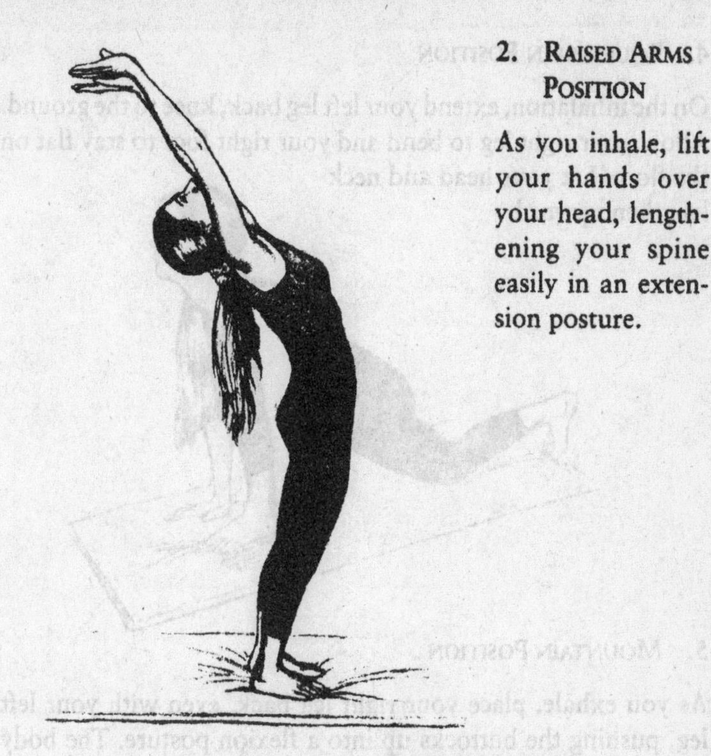

2. RAISED ARMS POSITION

As you inhale, lift your hands over your head, lengthening your spine easily in an extension posture.

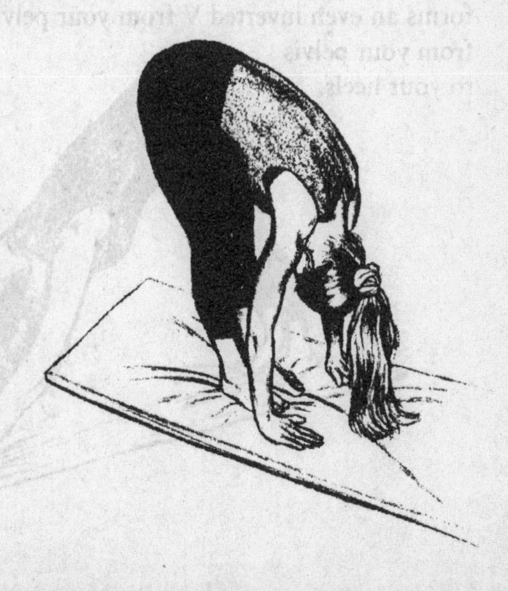

3. HAND TO FOOT POSITION

As you exhale, bend your body forward and down into a flexion posture. Allow your knees to bend.

4. Equestrian Position

On the inhalation, extend your left leg back, knee to the ground. Allow your right leg to bend and your right foot to stay flat on the floor. Let your head and neck lengthen upward.

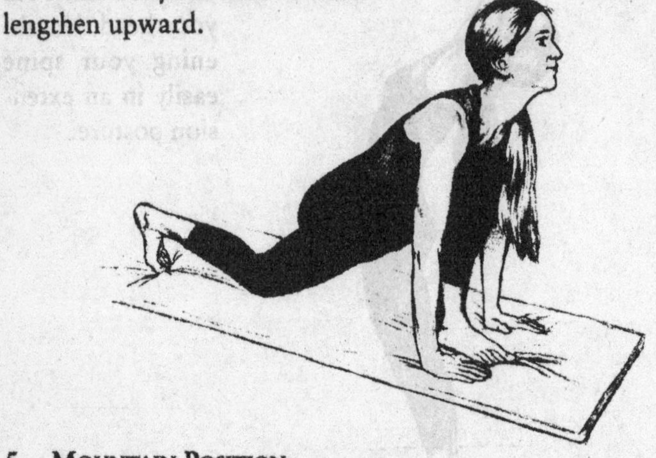

5. Mountain Position

As you exhale, place your right leg back, even with your left leg, pushing the buttocks up into a flexion posture. The body forms an even inverted V from your pelvis to your hands and from your pelvis to your heels.

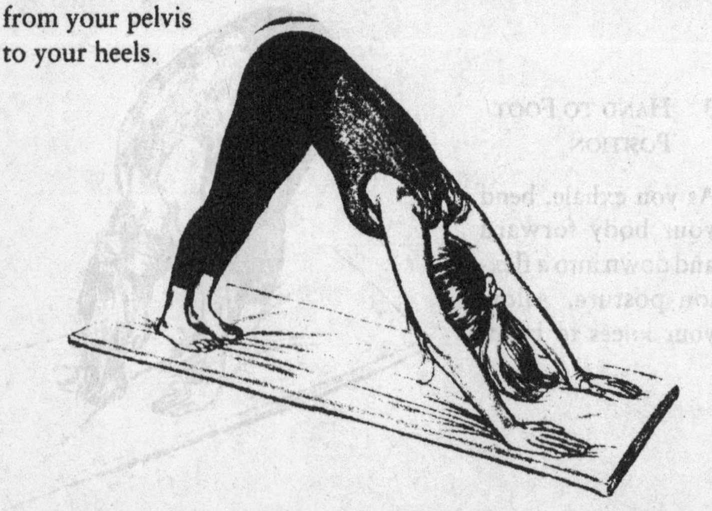

6. EIGHT LIMBS POSITION

Carefully drop both knees to the ground and allow your body to slide down at an angle, with your chest and chin briefly on the ground. Hold this briefly and then move smoothly into the next position.

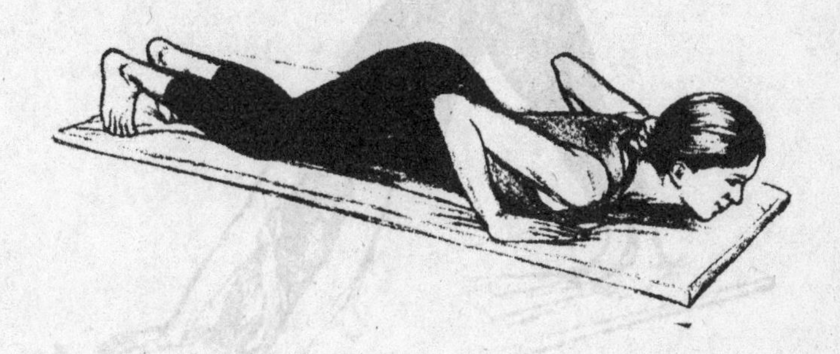

7. COBRA POSITION

As you inhale, lift your chest up and slightly forward while pressing down with your hands. Keep your elbows close to your body. Allow your spine to lift your head—do not start the movement with your head or lift your body with your neck.

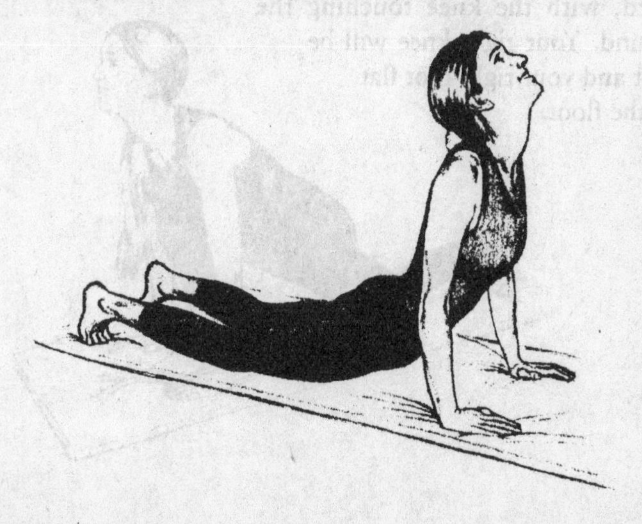

8. Mountain Position

While exhaling, raise your buttocks and hips in a flexion posture, the same as position 5.

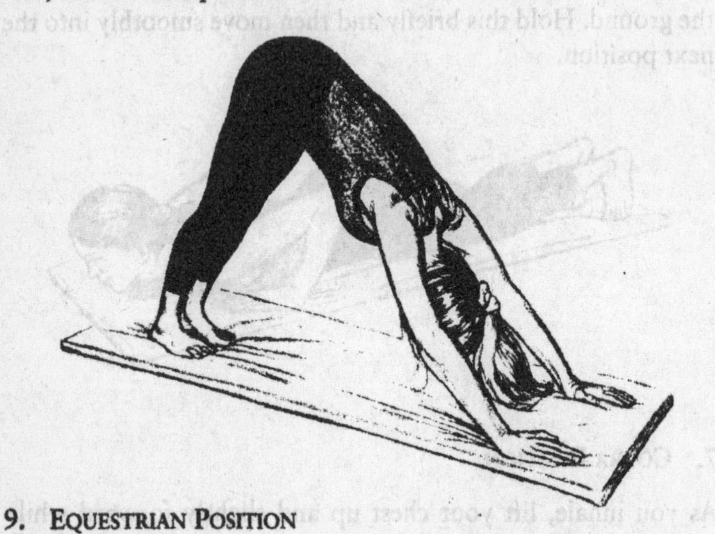

9. Equestrian Position

As you inhale, bring your right leg forward, between your hands, the same as position 4. Let your left leg extend backward, with the knee touching the ground. Your right knee will be bent and your right foot flat on the floor.

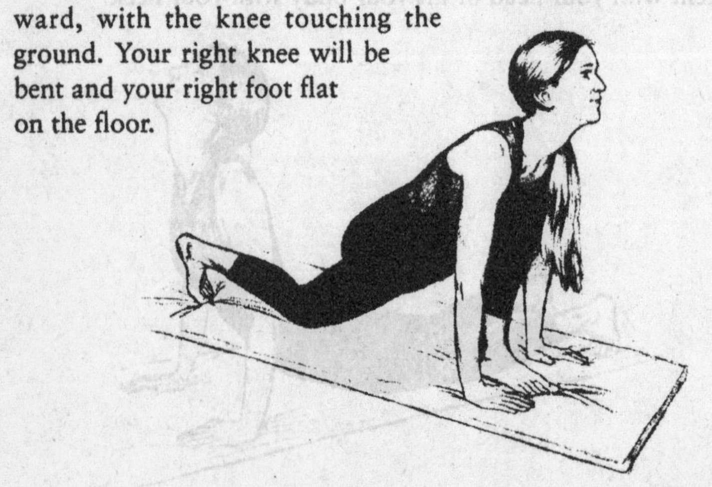

10. HAND TO FOOT POSITION

Repeat position 3. As you exhale, bend your body forward and down, coming down into a flexion posture. Allow your knees to bend.

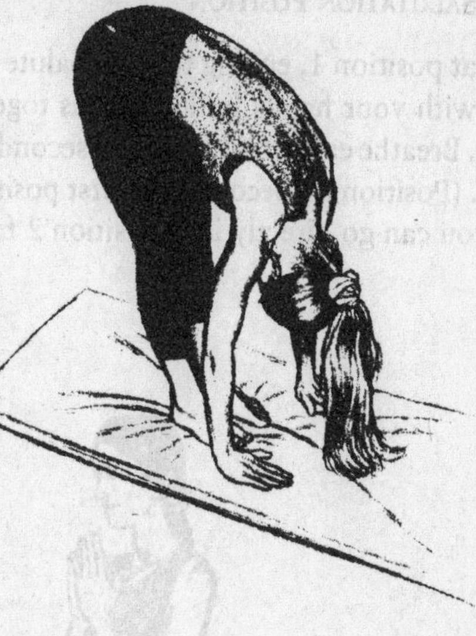

11. RAISED ARMS POSITION

Repeat position 2. As you inhale, lift your hands over your head, lengthening your spine easily in an extension posture.

12. Salutation Position

Repeat position 1, ending the Sun Salute the same way you began, with your hands folded, palms together, in front of your chest. Breathe easily for about five seconds. Then begin the next cycle. (Position 12 becomes the first position for the second cycle; you can go directly into position 2 from here.)

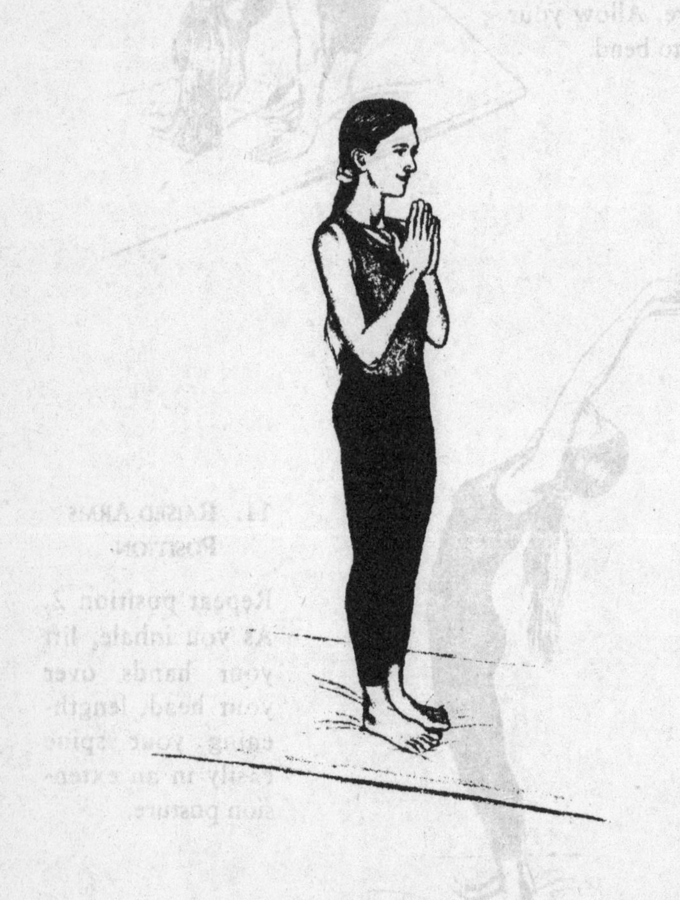

7

Chronic Fatigue in Today's Environment

The environment around us is a reflection of the collective consciousness of the population—this is a fundamental idea in Ayurvedic philosophy. For the past 150 to 200 years, however, society's prevailing view has been that humanity is separate from nature, and even superior to it. Man's role has been to subdue and exploit nature for his own material purposes. The result of this, as we are all now aware, has been scientific and industrial technologies that promote many forms of imbalance, including depletion of natural resources, pollution of air and water, and the possibility of major ecological disasters.

Fortunately, the pendulum has started to swing in the opposite direction. The collective consciousness of society is beginning to recognize that restoring balance to the natural environment is crucial for individual and global well-being. But while there is now reason for hope, we also need to recognize the negative effects that environmental disruptions are still inflicting, and how these can weaken health and drain energy.

If you are chronically tired, and no clear physical diagnosis has emerged to explain it, you should at least consider the possibility that aspects of your physical environment may be responsible for your diminished energy. The following Primary Energy Principle summarizes an important relationship that exists between every human being and his or her surroundings. Please write this down:

> PEP 18. Balance in the environment promotes balance in the individual; environmental imbalances can lead to individual imbalances.

Before we begin to explore these ideas, let me offer a word of caution. It is possible to become preoccupied by—or even obsessed with—the specter of environmental danger. Compulsive worrying about hazards in water, air, food, electromagnetic fields, and much more, can itself cause you to live in an unnatural and unhealthy condition. Such pervasive fear can bring about a greater physiological imbalance than would result from anything but the most dire environmental catastrophe. With this caution in mind, we can realistically assess some of the environmental influences that may be sources of chronic fatigue.

AIR QUALITY

Prana is the Ayurvedic term for air and breathing, but the word also has connotations of vitality, vital breath, and even of life itself. In addition to its fundamental importance in respiration, oxygen is one of the main components in the metabolism of food into vital energy. So the quality of the air we breathe obviously has great significance.

The most important Ayurveda principle in this area is the importance of getting fresh air every day. It's amazing how little fresh air many Americans get in their daily routine, and how draining this can be to vitality. Many people work in sealed environments where the flow of air is controlled by unseen fans or air conditioners. These cannot possibly provide the freshness that used to be available from open windows. People can now go for days or even weeks with only the slightest exposure to open air, especially during the winter months.

Fortunately, this is not a difficult situation to remedy. It's easy to create several opportunities each day for walking outdoors, even during the winter. Try getting off the bus a couple of stops before your destination, for instance, or park your car a few blocks away from your house or place of work. I recommend ten to fifteen minutes of fresh air once or twice every day. You'll feel immediate benefits in your vitality and sense of well-being.

It's also possible to bring more fresh air into indoor environments. Leave your windows open as much as possible during the warmer months, and in winter open your windows for at least ten minutes twice a day. Since you won't be able to do this if you work in a sealed glass-and-steel building, it will then be especially important to get outdoors for a walk at some point during the day, perhaps at lunchtime.

Air quality has improved in many urban areas during the past few years and one hopes this trend will continue. But if you suffer from significant chronic fatigue and you live in an area that is known to be badly polluted, you should be aware of the effects that air quality can have on your situation. It may be worthwhile to consider moving to a cleaner environment.

WATER QUALITY

Few people are aware of what's in the water they drink. While there's a perception that large cities have the most serious water-quality problems, some rural areas have comparable or even worse situations because of the effects of toxic chemicals in pesticides. If you are concerned about the quality of water in your area, you should contact your local water department or the district office of the Environmental Protection Agency for more information.

You can also take two simple measures for insuring purer drinking water. First, you can install a good-quality water filter in your home. The best filters are those that use reverse osmosis; they're called "RO" filters for short. A second approach is to drink and cook exclusively with bottled water. If you choose to do this, check the source of the water. Some "spring" water may not be pure, since many natural springs are now unfortunately contaminated by pollutants. A better option may be bottled filtered water, especially reverse osmosis–filtered.

FOOD QUALITY

We've already discussed the significance of fresh food and its vitalizing properties. In addition to freshness, it's important for food to be as free as possible from contaminants. All fruits and vegetables should of course be washed before eating, and you should also consider spending a little more to get produce that has been grown free of pesticides. Organically produced meats are also preferred, although environmental pollutants tend to concentrate in the tissues of all animals no matter how they're raised, and this is especially true in certain larger kinds of fish. There's also reason for concern about hormones given to livestock in order to increase bulk. All these factors make reduced consumption of meat and fish a wise choice.

MANMADE MATERIALS

Every day we come into contact with innumerable substances in the environment. In general, Ayurveda recommends emphasizing contact with natural substances and minimizing contact with artificially produced ones. This makes perfect sense biologically, because the human body evolved over thousands of years to interact with natural materials. Keep this principle in mind in constructing your home and work environments.

When you select clothing, be aware that cotton or wool allows your skin to breathe more freely than synthetics do. Linens and bedclothes should also be made of natural fabrics.

ELECTROMAGNETIC POLLUTION

There has been some attention in the media to the possible cancer-causing effects of cellular telephones, high-voltage transformers, microwave transmitters, computers, and other powerful sources of electrical energy. Research in this area is far from conclusive, and I caution you from becoming preoccupied with such concerns. But I do believe that prolonged exposure to electromagnetic forces in the environment can weaken the body and open the way for health problems. So if you're constantly or frequently in the presence of a known source of magnetic field radiation, you should be aware that this may be causing chronic fatigue. With regard to computers, it's probably a good idea to stay at least one arm's length away from the screen—and remember that more radiation is emitted from the sides, back, and top of a computer screen than through the front. I recommend you do some reading in this area in order to make an educated decision about the effect this may be having on your body.

Let me conclude this discussion of environmental hazards by emphasizing a positive point. The human body has a tremendous capacity for adjustment and self-repair, and there are many instances of this. The immune system, for example, is capable of recognizing and destroying almost every conceivable type of germ or biological invader, even ones it has never previously encountered. This remarkable degree of flexibility and self-protection is present in the body's detoxifying systems as well. By putting your attention on strengthening your body's own self-healing mechanisms, you can make yourself virtually invincible to many destructive influences. Though your environment may well contain pollutants, your system will be able to handle these to a large degree. At the same time, by checking your surroundings for any extreme instances of imbalance, you can take action to eliminate them and thereby maintain the strength of your body's natural self-repair processes.

BALANCE AND THE SENSES

The effects of the environment on human physiology are a function not only of what's "out there," but also of how we ourselves perceive and process the surrounding world. The five senses—hearing, touch, sight, taste, smell—are the five gateways through which we become aware of all environmental influences. If these senses are healthy and balanced, they naturally filter out many potentially harmful influences—and at the same time, they facilitate the acquisition of nourishment and energy.

Ultimately, balance of the senses depends upon balance of awareness and of consciousness. There is an ancient Ayurveda saying that expresses this truth: "The world is as we are." Please write it down as our next Primary Energy Principle:

> PEP 19. The world is as we are—our experience of the world depends upon the state of our awareness.

An analogy can illustrate this point. A day can be bright and sunny, but if you're wearing extremely dark sunglasses everything will look dismal and gray. If you now put on rose-colored glasses, everything will of course look rosy—and if you take your glasses off altogether, you'll suddenly realize the true beauty of the day. The way you experience the world depends just as much, or more, on the quality of your perceptions as it does on whatever is being perceived. If you are experiencing balance, creativity, and inner fulfillment, this is what you will find all around you.

I would like to look at the five senses in some detail, because bringing them into balance can reveal a whole new source of untapped energy within yourself.

One of the most important things to realize about the senses is the fact that they both give and receive information. On the one hand, they provide channels through which stimuli can flow from outside to inside. You can ingest and metabolize perceptions through your five senses in much the same way as you eat and digest food. And since assimilating information through the senses has a tremendous effect on the brain—and therefore on all the powerful neurochemicals that circulate throughout the body—it's important for your sensory influences to be nourishing and energy-producing, rather than toxic and energy-draining.

At the same time, the five senses are channels through which your awareness and your individual consciousness is projected outward to the world. This fact is often overlooked in modern physiology, but it is important in traditional health systems such as Ayurveda.

This projection of your inner intelligence can be a creative act that brings exhilaration and joy, or it can be a kind of empty hole into which your inner vitality flows and then disappears. Ayurveda teaches that the difference between these two possibilities depends on the extent to which you become entrapped by the object you're perceiving. If the sense of your own being and your own worth becomes identified with the object, you are experiencing "object-referral" rather than "self-referral." We'll discuss these very important concepts, and the whole mechanism of the senses as projectors of consciousness, in the the final chapter of this book.

For the balance of this chapter, we will be concerned with

the flow of information *inward* via the five senses to your individual awareness—and we'll explore what you can do to ensure that this inward flow is balanced and nourishing.

Before considering the senses individually, please write down this next Primary Energy Principle:

> PEP 20. The five senses are gateways to the mind/body system. By choosing sensory input that is harmonious and balancing, you can help cultivate happiness and energy throughout your system.

THE SENSE OF HEARING

The phrase "noise pollution" came into being several decades ago. It refers to the modern phenomenon of very loud or very unpleasant sound, and to the effect of such sound on the human beings who have to hear it. Physiologically speaking, noise pollution creates a kind of sensory hyperarousal. It is an excessive level of input to the nervous system that creates an alarmed response. If continued for more than a moment, it can cause a fight-or-flight response that is wearying to maintain. The end result of prolonged exposure to noise pollution, therefore, is chronic fatigue.

Noise is another environmental problem that may be difficult to resolve, especially if you live in a busy urban area. But there are creative ways to insulate yourself from noise pollution and to create a quieter, more harmonious environment. You can begin by relocating work or sleeping areas to the quietest part of an office or house, and you can use draperies and overstuffed furniture to muffle noise. Try some different options and see which work best for you. When you do have control over the kinds of sounds you're exposed to, make a conscious effort for them to be as pleasant and relaxing as possible.

I urge you to avoid loud, discordant music and to take advantage of the mind/body benefits of soothing musical sound. Research has shown that different harmonies and instrumental combinations can create different physiological effects. As the human physiology changes throughout the day under the cyclical influences of Vata, Pitta, and Kapha, particular sound values can help to maintain biological rhythms and to create overall balance. In this way, your sense of sound can be used for the well-being of your whole system.

There are certain key moments during each day when sound can have an especially important effect. By listening to soothing music at bedtime, for example, you can cultivate a natural state of serenity and restfulness. An entire branch of Ayurveda, called *gandhama veda*, is devoted to creating physiological balance through sound. Audiocassette selections of gandhama veda appropriate for bedtime may be ordered through Quantum Publications or other Ayurvedic sources whose addresses are provided at the end of this book. Simply play the cassette at low volume while you're lying down with the lights out.

THE SENSE OF TOUCH

During our discussion of the neuromuscular integration exercises, I mentioned marmas, points on the body similar to control switches through which energy is routed to various areas. Many of these vital points are located on the surface of your skin, and marma therapy is an aspect of Ayurveda that deals with balancing them. You can do a type of marma therapy at home that is very effective and which, in fact, you have already learned. It is the Ayurvedic oil massage described in chapter 5. This massage balances Vata throughout the system, and it does so by stimulating all the marma points on your skin's surface.

In addition to those on the skin, important marma points are on the scalp, the ears, and the soles of the feet, so I recommend that you spend a bit more time on these areas during your massage. Also, there are three other key marma points to which you should pay special attention, as they are the centers of Vata, Pitta, and Kapha. One is in the center of the forehead, another is near the lower part of the breastbone just over the heart, and the last is on the lower abdomen about two inches below the navel. Using gentle pressure, simply make a large circular motion over each of these three areas during your massage; traditionally, a clockwise motion is recommended.

Giving attention to the marma points on your skin through the daily oil massage will help to awaken integrated energy flow throughout your body.

THE SENSE OF SIGHT

Of all the senses, sight provides the greatest volume of perceptual information. It is also the one most subject to sensory overload. A tired feeling around the eyes, headaches, and twitches of the eye muscles are all indicators of this overloading, which can be a major energy drain. Most of the recommendations for dealing with this are rather obvious; you shouldn't read in dim light, for example. But you should also be alert to sensory overload through your eyes just as we discussed in connection with hearing and noise pollution. For most people, this problem originates with excessive exposure to movies and television. Indeed, a great deal of visual entertainment is a kind of intentional sensory overload, and it can be a significant drain on your energy level.

Try taking a few nights off from watching television, then use your Energy Tracking Chart to note how you feel during the following days. Many people experience greater balance, calm, and centeredness, which translates into increased energy throughout the day. Occasional TV or a movie can certainly be enjoyable, but if you've developed a dependency on these media you should be aware of their energy-depleting effects.

THE SENSE OF TASTE

As we discussed in connection with diet, the most important point concerning taste is to experience all six tastes every day, and ideally at every meal. This not only improves digestion and helps balance your system, it adds zest to your whole experience of life.

In general, the following common spices are recommended for use in cooking or at the table: black pepper, ginger, rock salt (if available), cumin, turmeric, cardamom, cinnamon, cloves, and mustard seeds. All these spices are considered to have sattvic, or energizing, qualities. Hot spices such as cayenne pepper and chilis should be used sparingly or not at all, especially by Pitta types.

THE SENSE OF SMELL

Ayurveda considers the sense of smell to have a particularly potent effect on the mind/body system. We all know the power of smell to evoke memories and emotions: how walking into a room and encountering a certain fragrance can instantly call up vivid memories of the distant past. This is because the olfactory nerve carries its information directly to the deepest regions of the brain, where emotion and many of the body's most basic functions are regulated.

The use of scent or aroma to create physiological balance is an ancient part of classical Ayurveda. Certain scents have influences on particular doshas, and in general the pattern is similar to that of the tastes. Sweet or sour scents tend to balance

Vata dosha, for example, while spicy fragrances balance Kapha, and minty scents balance Pitta. Aromatic oils for balancing the doshas are available through sources listed at the end of this book. The best way to use aromas is at bedtime in order to create a fragrance that will last through the night. The Vata aroma is usually recommended for this purpose, since pacifying or balancing Vata is conducive to sleep. During the daytime, you may also find aroma therapy to be particularly balancing and enlivening. Choose an aroma in the same way you might choose your body-type diet for a given day, based on an awareness of the leading doshas in your physiology and on the season of the year.

8

Joy as the Foundation of Energy

Although biological factors are certainly important in overcoming chronic fatigue, it should also be obvious that human life requires something more than proper nutrition and exercise in order to be really healthy. There must be a sense of meaning, an awareness of some larger purpose, a focus on some worthwhile goal.

One of the most intriguing insights of traditional Ayurveda is expressed in the following Primary Energy Principle. Please write this down:

PEP 21. Growth is the foundation of survival.

In this context, survival does not mean simply staying alive and continuing to breathe. It means living in a spiritually meaningful way. One can avoid biological death by eating and drinking some minimal amount every twenty-four hours, but in order to live in any true sense of the word there must be progress and growth. The alternative is stagnation, chronic fatigue, or an even more serious imbalance.

Spiritual growth is an exhilarating experience. It sustains us emotionally through the ups and downs of life, and it is biologically important as well. A sense of progress and direction in your life fosters creation of the neurochemicals that can energize and vitalize your entire mind/body system. This is the real key to dynamic energy.

WHOLENESS AND CONNECTION

The spiritual growth I'm speaking of here is simply the unfolding and fulfillment of human potential. Within you is the impulse to be the very best you can possibly be—but there's something even more than that. Deep down, everyone suspects that he or she has the potential to be truly great. Greatness is—or at least *was* at some time—the real goal of every person's life.

In children the impulse to be great can be clearly seen. Children have no doubts about their ability to achieve what they want, and to be exactly who they want to be. In everything they do there is joy and spontaneity—and unbounded energy as well.

What word can we use to describe this state of being? It is a state of completely experiencing every moment to the very limit. It is a *wholeness* of being.

The impulse to wholeness is a natural human birthright, for within each of us there is the possibility of wholeness and the deep desire to achieve it. Wholeness means being completely integrated, without any sense of being separate, fragmented, or limited. It means experiencing natural joy.

In Ayurveda, this wholeness has traditionally been seen as the goal of human development. Modern psychologists have referred to it as a state of "self-actualization." As originally described by the psychologist Abraham Maslow, self-actualization is characterized by creativity, a sense of inner freedom, fulfillment, energy, and spontaneity. Maslow felt that this state is a natural goal in the evolution of every person.

Wholeness and self-actualization is something that many people have spontaneously felt, at least for brief periods in their lives. It may have come in sports, in a particularly rewarding experience in your work, or in a moment shared with another person. Regardless of the specifics, these beautiful occasions are invariably accompanied by joy, by a sense of everything flowing effortlessly, and by a feeling of intimate connection with other people and with the larger environment.

Ayurveda has long seen this sense of connection as a basic truth that every person should strive to realize—and now modern science is also telling us that we are indeed intimately connected to all of nature and to the source of energy itself. Perhaps the greatest benefit of Ayurveda lies in its highly practical techniques for balancing our mind/body systems and thereby reestablishing our links with the true wellsprings of vitality and health.

TEACHING YOURSELF TO GO BEYOND

I urge you to consider this vision of wholeness in the context of your own life. Over the years, many of us develop attitudes and self-concepts that diminish the unlimited sense of potential we enjoyed as children. Delays, frustrations, and defeats inevitably occur, and these give rise to second thoughts about the possibility of fulfilling our goals.

Ayurveda states that three experiences—rejection, disappointment, and doubt—are the most dangerous creators of stress in the system. As a result of these painful experiences, we can develop attitudes that are self-limiting rather than self-expanding. At first, these defensive feelings may have quite understandably developed as a way of protecting the heart from further disappointments, but the effect of such self-limitation is nonetheless devastating for spiritual growth.

Here I have in mind such destructive thoughts as: *"I guess I'll never be completely happy, but who's really happy anyway?"; "I guess I'll never achieve my goals, but they were probably unrealistic"; "I'm not the kind of person who can really be successful in anything."*

I can hardly imagine any phrase more self-limiting than "I'm not the kind of person who..."!

The most dangerous aspect of these negative attitudes is the way they come to be reflected in the neurochemistry of our bodies. Because the mind/body connection is always at work, destructive thinking eventually translates into some destructive physical condition such as chronic fatigue. Fatigue, after all, is really just a kind of inertia, a physical sense of disappointment with life.

The key to overcoming these pessimistic, soul-shrinking attitudes is to go beyond them through the unlimited spiritual power that really is within you, though you may have lost sight of it for the moment. Going beyond is the only way. This is something more than just positive thinking; it's gaining access to a deeper level of organizing power, a stronger force for coherence. What I mean by "going beyond" is getting to the source of thought, and reaching the unified field of pure joy and unlimited possibility.

The breathing meditation technique presented in chapter 5 is one of the most effective methods for accomplishing this. The classical textbooks of Ayurveda clearly describe the benefits of incorporating meditation into your daily activity: when you emerge from the meditation period, some of the unboundedness and inner potential you experienced while meditating will stay with you. One could put it in neuropsychological terms by saying that the brain wave integration that takes place during the practice of meditation persists into other activities. New circuits, new areas of the brain become available to you for the first time for your thoughts, perceptions, and actions.

Reaching the source of thought is also, of course, an experience of reaching your own inner being; it's the most profound kind of self-realization. Many people describe this as "coming back home" or "discovering who I really am."

Through breathing meditation and the other techniques presented in this book, you can again contact your vast inner potential, perhaps for the first time since you were a child. You can reestablish the connection between your own individual self and the unbounded energy and creativity of nature.

OBJECT-REFERRAL VS. SELF-REFERRAL

As you begin to function more and more from within yourself, your self-concept inevitably becomes less and less dependent on the opinions of others. In Ayurveda, this is called becoming "self-referral" instead of "object-referral."

Object-referral means sacrificing your unique inner identity for the sake of an externally manufactured self-image. It means defining yourself in terms of what others might be thinking. Everything you do must be carefully plotted out, all your energy is directed outward toward some object or person, and this is very fatiguing. In Ayurveda, this is called *pragyaparadh*, the mistaken intellect. The mind makes the mistake of thinking that its true nature depends upon things outside itself.

In contrast, self-referral means locating your true identity and meaningfulness within yourself. There's no impulse to deliberately calculate actions and appearances; they are just intuitively and spontaneously *right*. At the silent level of the mind, at the deepest level of your nature, there is a computing system far more reliable than any conscious plans or thoughts. By gaining access to nature's inner, effortless computing system, you liberate huge amounts of energy and creativity. Fatigue is suddenly a thing of the past.

PRESENT-MOMENT AWARENESS

Self-referral awareness is present-moment awareness. Life is spontaneously organized by experiencing the present, rather than by ruminating on the past or worrying about the future. But object-referral awareness is based on fear and worry. This is because the object of attention is always changing—and who can predict the opinions of others, much less the flow of external events? Object-referral is invariably a fear-based way of life, and nothing dissipates energy sooner than fear.

Our next Primary Energy Principle sums up the ideas we've discussed so far in this chapter. Please write this down:

> PEP 22. Wholeness of life is the goal of individual human growth and evolution. Wholeness is self-referral rather than object-referral, is centered in present-moment awareness, and is characterized by inner freedom, creativity, spontaneity, and nature's unlimited energy.

DHARMA

In Ayurveda there is an important concept concerning individual human evolution, which is the notion of dharma. Dharma may be translated as one's natural path, natural behavior, or natural duty. It refers to the fact that everyone has a course of action that is most right and nourishing for him or her, a path that creates greatest happiness and speediest evolution.

There are two aspects to dharma: one is universal, the other individual. Everyone has a universal dharma, which is to achieve wholeness of life. This is built into the mind/body system; it is inscribed in our DNA. Each generation inherits an inner impulse to grow from the previous generation. We all possess this drive to achieve full potential, both mentally and physically. In physical terms, this means achieving perfect health. Emotionally and psychologically, it means gaining that state of stability, creativity, and bliss that we've called self-actualization or self-realization. Ayurveda calls this "enlightenment."

Along with this universal dharma, there is also an individual dharma. This is the course of action that is most appropriate for each human being and will help to bring him or her more quickly to the goal of wholeness of life. For certain people, being an airline pilot or an army general may provide just the right opportunity for growth. Others may need to be homemakers or teachers. But if the action is truly dharmic, in every case it feels right; it feels natural; and it produces happiness.

Individual dharma can change with the passage of time. For example, it is dharmic for most people to be unmarried while growing up and attending school, but later the dharma for most is family life. Occupational interests and even lifestyle orientations may change at different times of life, as one completes one phase of dharma and enters another.

Above all, dharma is meant to be a vehicle for the unfolding of happiness, wholeness, and health. If a certain action is right and natural—if it is in the direction of evolution—the mind/body system will experience a sense of comfort, satisfaction, and even bliss in the performance of that action. But if an activity impedes the evolutionary path, this will be expressed as physical and emotional discomfort, which very often takes the form of chronic fatigue.

How should you go about finding your dharma? At the outset, it's very important to recognize that universal dharma and individual dharma nourish and support each other. If you're confused about what your individual dharma may be, you should direct attention to developing your universal dharma—

to developing self-referral and wholeness. All the procedures and techniques in this book will help you to establish balance in mind and body. They will put you more in touch with your own inner resources of creativity and intelligence. With this broader perspective and enhanced creativity, you will naturally start to find greater satisfaction in your life. You'll recognize the most evolutionary, creative opportunities in every situation, and you'll be able to make the most of them. In the process of growth, you may even conclude that certain things ought to change, perhaps in your line of work or in some of your relationships. But the change will be natural, based on the broader perspective and greater creativity you're now able to bring to your situation. Your actions will be more and more in tune with your inner nature and with your individual dharma.

THE RECREATIONAL UNIVERSE

Along with life's work and duty, recreation is everyone's dharma. In fact, we live in a recreational universe. Just look around and you'll see that this is true: birds burst into song in the morning, porpoises leap through the waves, and everywhere joy is displayed in nature. Recreation is an intrinsic aspect of wholeness, and allowing enough time for recreation is an important part of growing toward that goal.

In connection with alleviating chronic fatigue, you should probably increase the amount of time you devote to recreation. Actually, I would describe many of the techniques in this book as recreational, including meditation, the Sun Salute, and neuromuscular-neurorespiratory integration techniques. Recreation, after all, literally means "*re*-creation": to rejuvenate and revitalize, to renew the body's resources and vital energy.

As an important part of a balanced life, Ayurveda definitely recommends taking at least one full day each week off from work. This day should be devoted completely to rest and recreation. Your mind/body system needs one full day each week free from the responsibilities of everyday life in order to renew and rejuvenate itself.

Our final Primary Energy Principle summarizes the main points about dharma. Please write it down:

> PEP 23. Dharma means a path of action that is the most right, evolutionary, and nourishing for your unique nature. Dharma has a universal aspect, which is the impulse to grow and to achieve wholeness of life, and an individual aspect, which includes the specific activities that are most appropriate and evolutionary for you as an individual.

BEHAVIORAL RASAYANAS

Ayurveda recognizes that certain actions are inherently nurturing to the human body and spirit. These are known as "behavioral rasayanas." They strengthen the physiology and replenish energy, because behavior that is positive and uplifting creates neurochemical changes that have beneficial effects on your own system.

When you project a behavior onto another person, for example, you yourself experience the results of that behavior, whether positive or negative. In Ayurveda, this has traditionally been thought of as the law of karma, but the idea also has a neurophysiological basis. In a very real sense, the effects of all your actions are manifested in your own good health, or lack of it.

Behavioral rasayanas are those actions that express respect, service, compassion, tolerance, and love. Respecting elders or teachers, supporting a person in need, spending time with learned people—these are some of the traditional behavioral rasayanas. But I believe the essence of the whole concept can be summed up in one sentence: *Favor the positive in every situation, and do not entertain negativity.*

I assure you that if you begin to apply this principle in your daily life, the first beneficiary of this practice will be you. The best time to use it is when you notice some level of physical or emotional discomfort, such as chronic fatigue, and you feel that your actions toward another person may be contributing to this. Immediately see if you can find something positive in the situation toward which you can shift your attention. And remember that placing your attention on something helps that thing to grow stronger. You'll be amazed how quickly most negative situations can be turned around by shifting your attention, and how exhilarated you'll feel as a result.

The other half of this principle is "not to entertain negativity," and here I think the word *entertain* is extremely important. No one can completely avoid the negative aspects of life, but there's no necessity to *entertain* them, either. If someone you don't like arrives uninvited at your home, you don't have to provide a comfortable environment for that person. Just ignore him and he'll soon leave on his own. In the same way, you don't have to dwell on pessimistic thoughts or black moods. The best attitude is indifference, together with a positive shift in awareness. With time, this refusal to entertain negativity will become easier and easier. And once again, meditation can be a great help in culturing the habit of positive thinking in a natural and effortless way.

All the principles and techniques you've encountered in this book are designed to help you achieve the state of balance that will hasten your progress on the path to fulfillment. To escape from self-limiting and fear-based attitudes and behaviors into the pure joy of self-referral and wholeness is to personally experience nature's boundless energy. It is permanently to replace fatigue with energy. And it is an important step toward ultimate wholeness, which is the true goal of your evolution as a human being.

BIBLIOGRAPHY

Bell, Davis S. *Curing Fatigue*. Emmaus, Penn.: Rodale Press, 1993.

Frawley, Dr. David, and Lad, Dr. Vasant. *The Yoga of Herbs*. Twin Lakes, Wis.: Lotus Press, 1986.

Hoffman, Ronald. *Tired All the Time*. New York: Poseidon Press, 1993.

Kapoor, L. D. *Handbook of Ayurveda Medicinal Plants*. Boca Raton, Fl.: CRC Press, 1990.

Rosenbaum, Michael, and Susser, Murray. *Solving the Problem of Chronic Fatigue Syndrome*. Tacoma, Wash.: Life Sciences Press, 1992.

Index

Deepak Chopra and The Chopra Center for Well Being in La Jolla, California, offer a wide range of seminars, products and educational programmes, worldwide. The Chopra Center offers revitalizing mind/body programmes, as well as day spa services. Guests can come to rejuvenate, expand knowledge or obtain a medical consultation.

For information on meditation classes, health and well-being courses, instructor certification programmes, or local classes in your area, contact The Chopra Center for Well Being, 7630 Fay Avenue, La Jolla, California, 92037, USA. By telephone: 001-888-424-6772, or 001-619-551-7788. For a virtual tour of the Center, visit the Internet website at www.chopra.com.

If you live in Europe and would like more information on workshops, lectures or other programmes about Dr. Deepak Chopra or to order any of his books, tapes or products, please contact: Contours, 44 Fordbridge Road, Ashford, Middlesex, TW15 2SJ (tel: +44 (0) 208 564 7033; fax: +44 (0) 208 897 3807; email: sales@infinite-contours.co.uk; website: www.infinite-contours.co.uk).

If you have enjoyed this book and would like the opportunity to explore higher realms of consciousness and have a more direct experience of divinity, you may do so interactively at Deepak Chopra's new website, www.mypotential.com.